Immunosuppression

Edited by Xuehui He

Published in London, United Kingdom

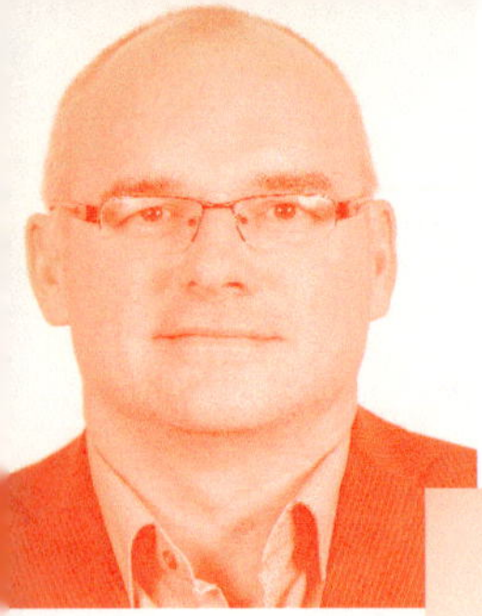
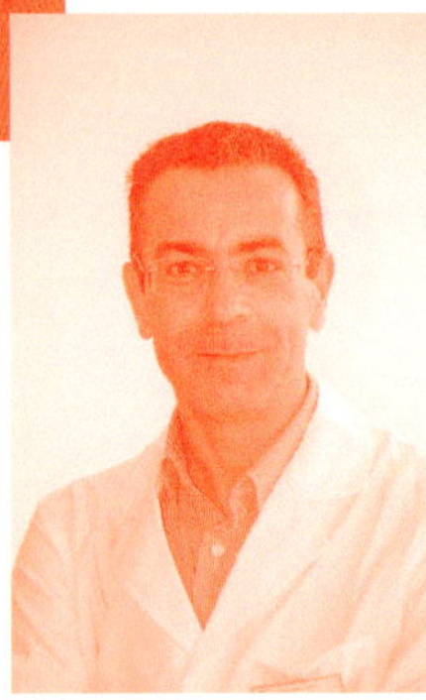
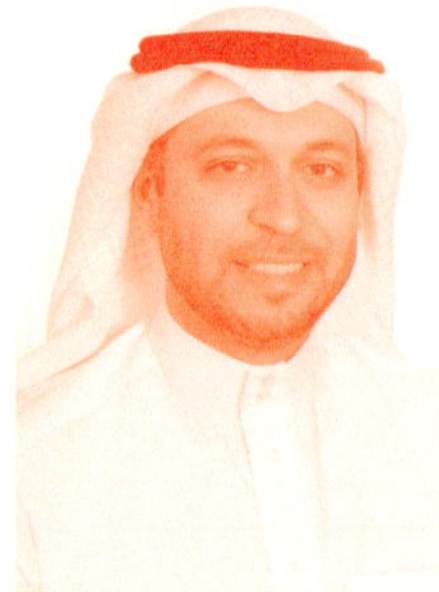
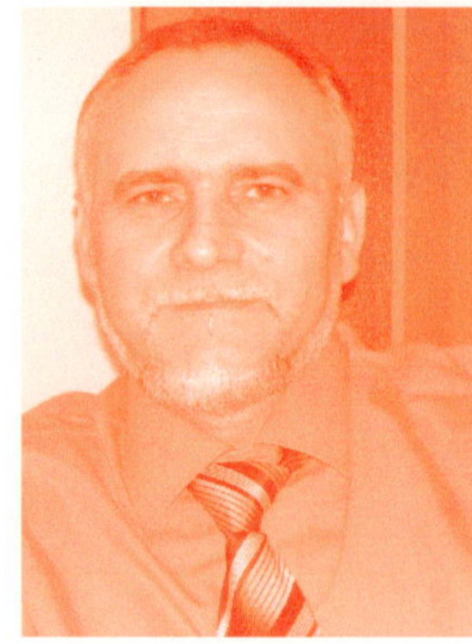
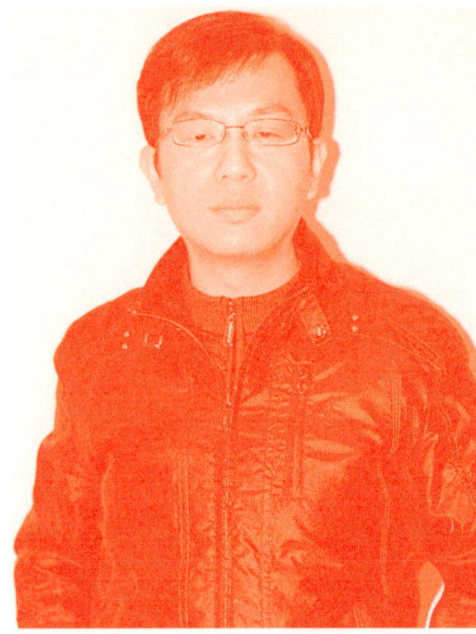
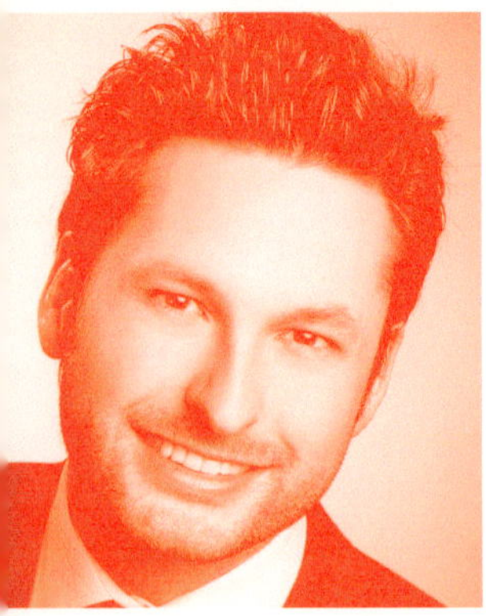
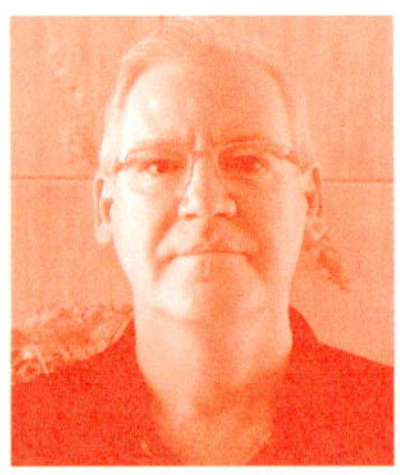

IntechOpen

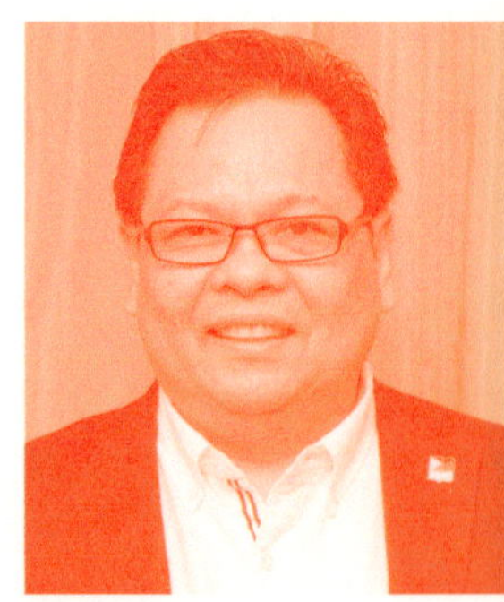
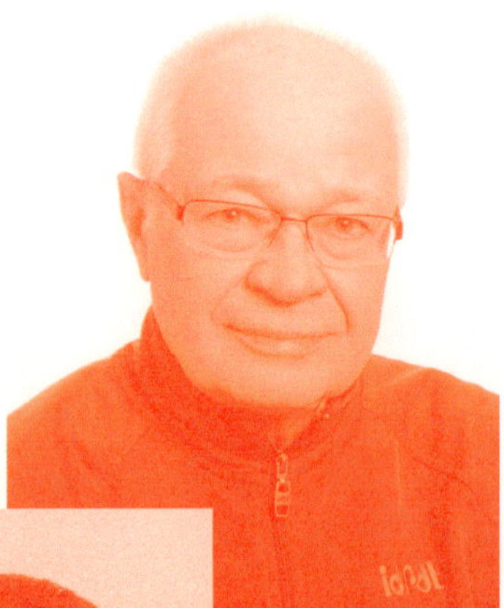
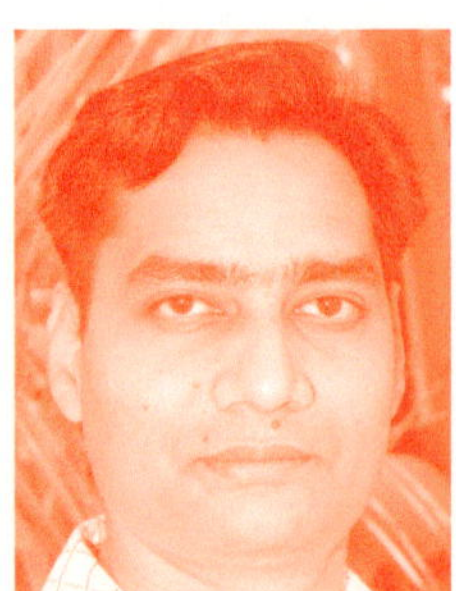
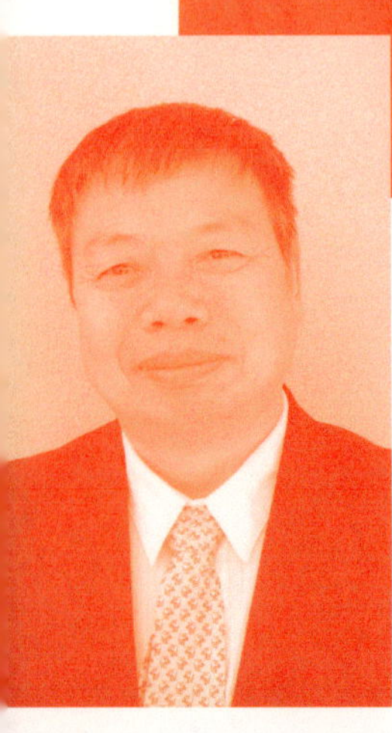
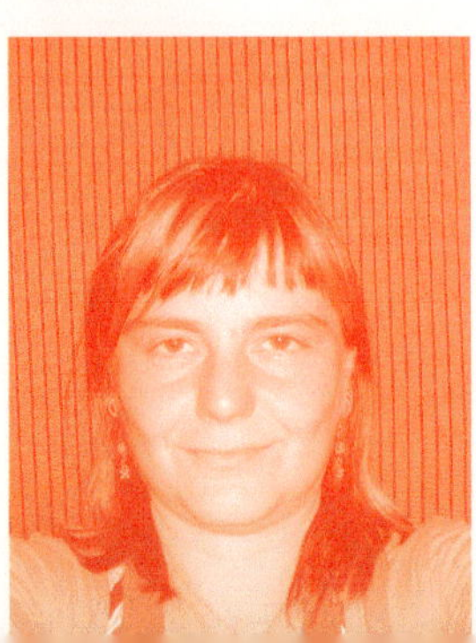
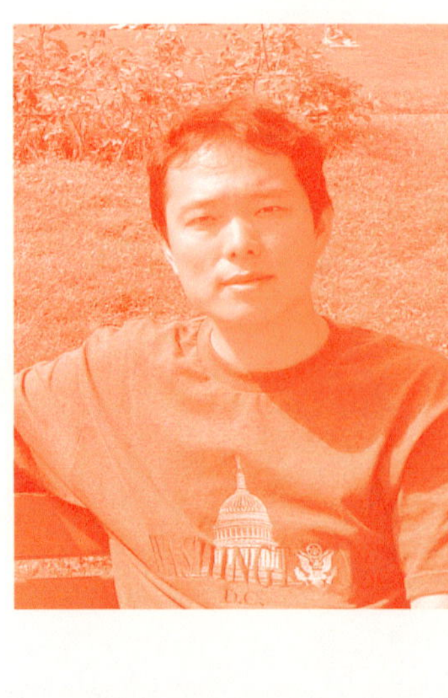

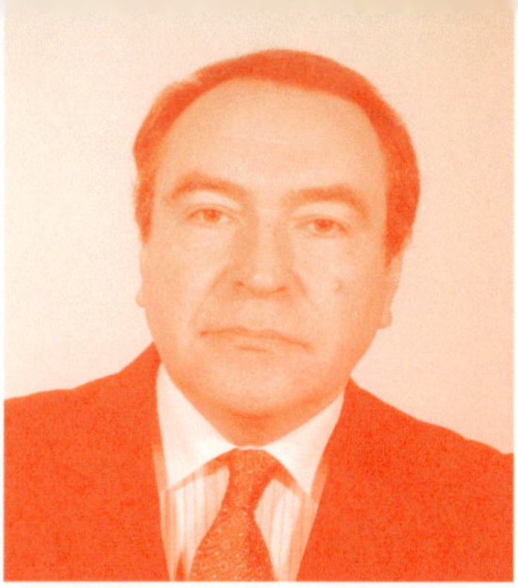

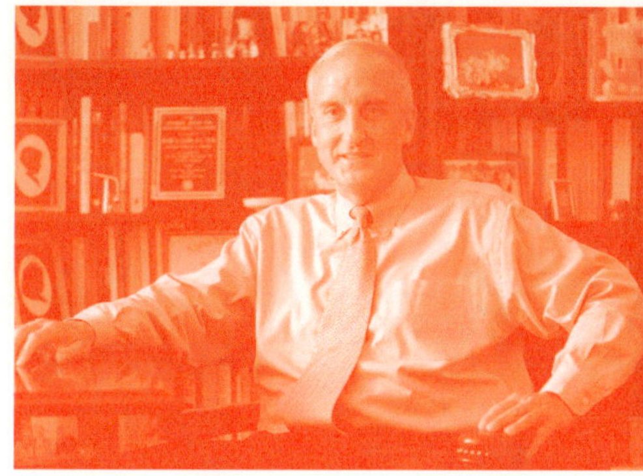

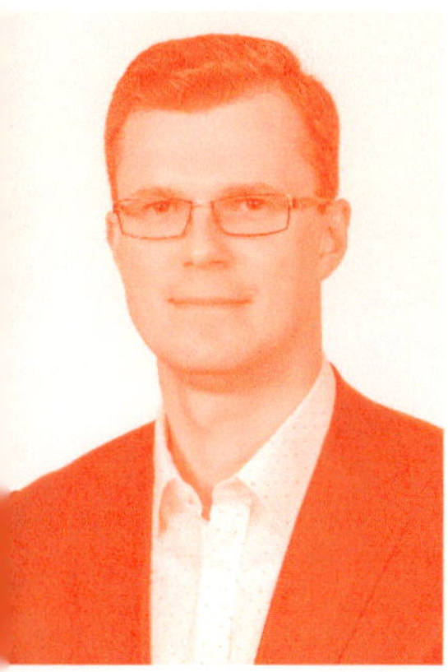

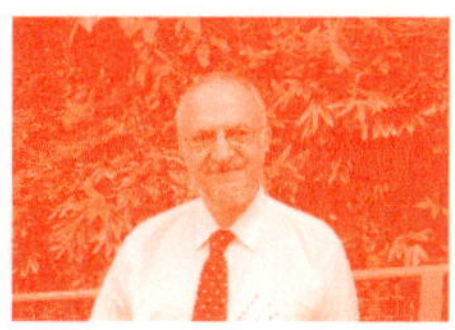

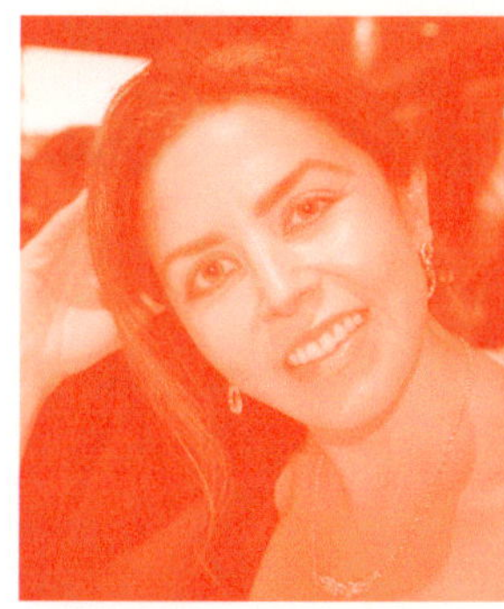

Supporting open minds since 2005

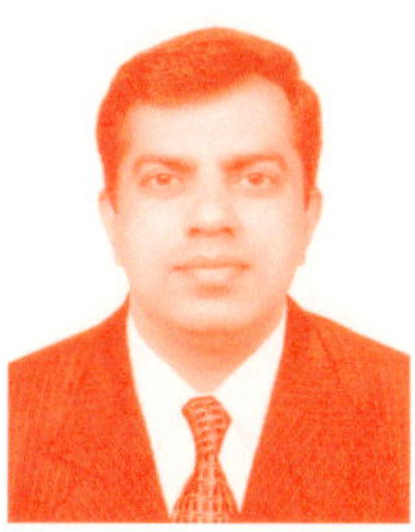

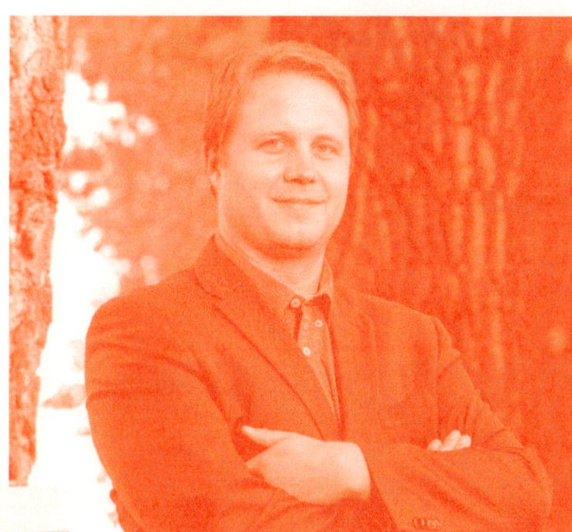

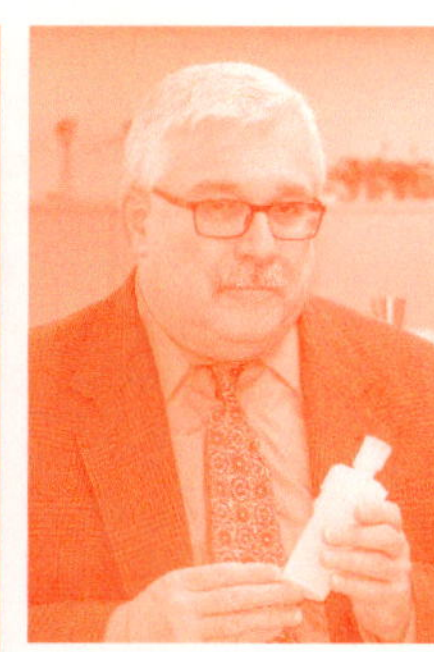

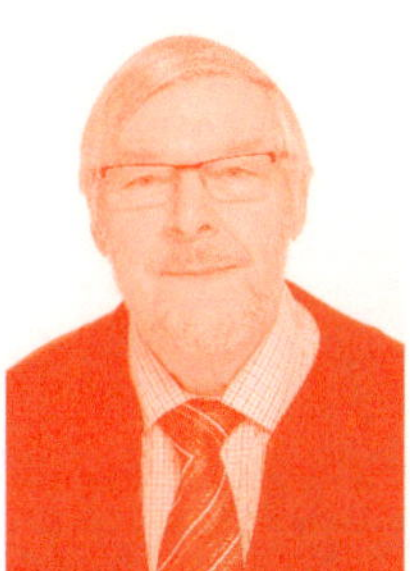

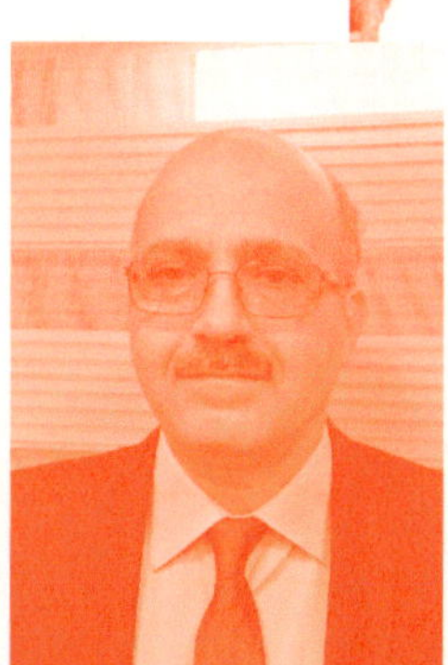

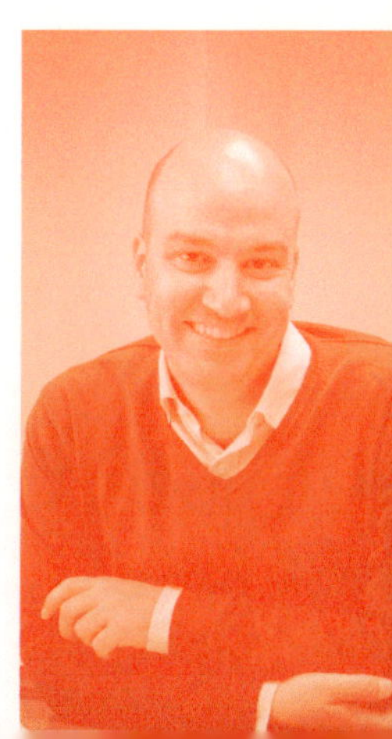

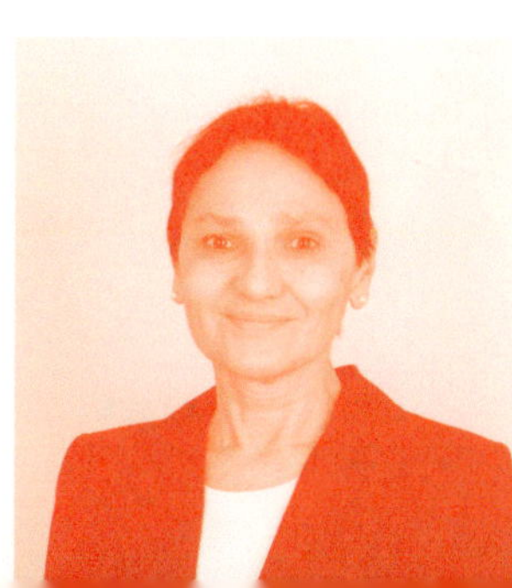

Immunosuppression
http://dx.doi.org/10.5772/intechopen.87403
Edited by Xuehui He

Contributors
Calvin S.H. Ng, Evan Qize Yuan, Evgeny Grigoryev, Vera Matveeva, Artem Ivkin, Maryam Khanova, Mark D. Scott, Xining Yang, Seema Naik, Kevin Rakszawski, Joseph Cioccio, Hiroko Shike, Hong Zheng, Takuya Watanabe, Norihide Fukushima, Cosmas Rinaldi A Lesmana, Kirana Mandasari

First published in London, United Kingdom, 2020 by IntechOpen
IntechOpen is the global imprint of INTECHOPEN LIMITED, registered in England and Wales, registration number: 11086078, 5 Princes Gate Court, London, SW7 2QJ, United Kingdom
Printed in Croatia

British Library Cataloguing-in-Publication Data
A catalogue record for this book is available from the British Library

Additional hard and PDF copies can be obtained from orders@intechopen.com

Immunosuppression
Edited by Xuehui He
p. cm.
Print ISBN 978-1-83968-123-3
Online ISBN 978-1-83968-124-0
eBook (PDF) ISBN 978-1-83968-125-7

For EU product safety concerns:
IN TECH d.o.o., Prolaz Marije Krucifikse Kozulić 3, 51000 Rijeka, Croatia, info@intechopen.com or visit our website at intechopen.com.

Meet the editor

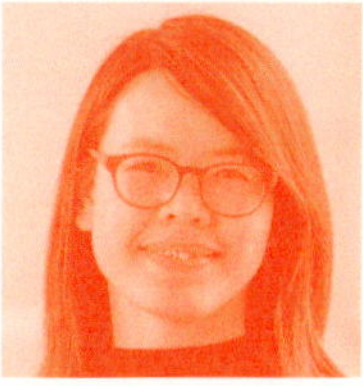

Dr. Xuehui He received her PhD at Tuebingen University, Germany, in the field of molecular biology. Thereafter, she moved to Nijmegen, The Netherlands, and started her adventure in the field of immunology. Over the years, the regulation of the immune system in relation to autoimmune diseases has been her main topic of research including the basics of T cell activation, the induction of immune tolerance, and the modulatory effect of various immune suppressants. Identification of biomarkers for personalized therapy and using the biomarker profile as a co-diagnostic tool is her recent research focus. Her final aim is to capture disease severity in validated outcome measures and assess side effects of treatments in real clinical practice.

Contents

Preface

To safeguard ourselves, our immune system is equipped with a series of defence mechanisms to recognise and respond to non-self molecules. Although essential for fighting off infections and preventing cancers, destructive immune responses pose a considerable challenge in autoinflammation and transplantation. Currently available immunosuppressants help to control destructive immune responses. However, management of side-effects of lifelong immunosuppression, including cancer development and reduced survival, remain major problems. For this reason, an increasing amount of interest is directed towards the natural specific regulatory mechanism of the immune system. A better understanding of these mechanisms holds the key.

One approach that the immune system employs to induce self-tolerance is via regulatory T cells (Treg). Treg are well known for their immune regulatory potential and are essential for maintaining immune homeostasis. Impaired Treg-mediated immune regulation has been observed in various autoimmune diseases as well as in cancers. Therefore, Treg might provide an ideal therapeutic target for diseases where the immune balance is impaired and could benefit from the regulation of Treg properties. The rationale of Treg-based immunotherapy for treating autoimmunity and transplant rejection is to tip the immune balance of effector T cell-mediated immune activation and Treg-mediated immune inhibition in favour of Treg cells, either through endogenous Treg expansion strategies or adoptive transfer of ex vivo expanded Treg. Human Treg are currently intensively studied for the induction of immunotolerance both in transplantation and autoimmunity. The tumour microenvironment preferably recruits immune cells, which possess a highly immunosuppressive capacity, thus inducing peripheral immune tolerance and facilitating tumour immune escape. Immune checkpoint inhibitors take the brakes off an immune response that has begun thus reactivating the anti-cancer effect.

In this book on immunosuppression, researchers in this area discuss their recent findings in the context of autoimmune diseases as well as cancers. Topics include biological modulation of Treg, monitoring of the complement pathway in the occurrence of antibody-mediated organ rejection, immunotherapy for bile duct cancer, immunosuppression in viral infections, and the management of biliary diseases using endoscopic ultrasound. These reviews are representative of a current active research field that continues to grow and enlighten. We hope the reviews will be of use to experts in the field and new entrants alike.

Dr. Xuehui He
Department of Laboratory Medicine,
Medical Immunology Section,
Radboud University,
Nijmegen, Netherlands

Chapter 1

Induced Immunosuppression in Critical Care

Evgeny Grigoryev, Vera Matveeva, Artem Ivkin and Maryam Khanova

Abstract

The maladaptive nature of the systemic inflammatory response syndrome, which may be caused by sepsis, trauma, or ischemia-reperfusion injury, is characterized by a shift towards the distant effects of pro- and anti-inflammatory mediators. Shock, blood loss, and metabolic disorders may cause the onset of multiple organ dysfunction syndrome. The final phase of critical illness is generally associated with induced immunosuppression and dysfunctions of neutrophils, monocytes and macrophages, dendritic cells, release of myeloid-derived suppressor cells, damage to glycocalyx and endothelium, and impaired metabolic conjugation. This review is aimed at providing novel evidences on the roles of various immune components, either innate or acquired, in the induction of immunosuppression from the standpoint of the rapid diagnosis of immune disorders in the intensive care unit using flow cytometry as a commonly accepted option.

Keywords: systemic inflammatory response syndrome, persistent multiple organ dysfunction, induced immunosuppression, flow cytometry

1. Introduction

Systemic inflammatory response syndrome (SIRS) refers to a critical illness, either infectious (sepsis) or secondary to tissue injury (tissue injury, cardiopulmonary bypass) that evolves into two phases. The first phase is an initial hyperinflammatory response, sometimes referred as a cytokine storm. Damage-associated molecular patterns (DAMP), also known as alarmins, and pathogen-associated molecular patterns (PAMP) activate the innate immune system. The activation of innate immunity is accompanied by a significant release of pro-inflammatory mediators that increase the intensity of the immune response and trigger adaptive immunity responses [1].

Excessive activation of pro-inflammatory mechanisms in SIRS patients drives the development of compensatory mechanisms to prevent excessive inflammation and weaken its excessive activity [2]. Negative feedback mechanisms downregulate this response in the first hours but may lead to the dysregulation and pathological over time, resulting in persistent suppression of immune response and increasing the risk of recurrent infections [3]. Numerous clinical and experimental trials on SIRS and sepsis have reported significant changes in the immunological profile, suggesting the phase of immune suppression to be the predominant immunological response in most patients after 7–14 days of persistent critical illness [4]. From the standpoint of critical care medicine, patients with sepsis cannot overcome the

IntechOpen

primary bacterial infection even if they are actively treated, including antibacterial therapy. Patients with SIRS- and sepsis-induced immunosuppression acquire nosocomial and opportunistic infections contributing to the onset of multiple organ dysfunction syndrome [5].

The development of MODS is propagated by the dysregulation of the immune system. However, the interplay of pathophysiological mechanisms underlying the dysregulation of immune inflammatory processes is complex and requires in-depth studies. These mechanisms and their role are changing during the progression of the disease implying a heterogeneous immunological status specific to each patient. To date, researchers have focused on understanding the main changes in the innate and adaptive cellular immunity in critically ill patients, which may aid in the development of early and accurate individualized therapy protocols. Therefore, flow cytometry may be considered as a promising tool, enabling collecting highly accurate data at the preanalytical stage within a relatively short period of time. This review summarizes and discusses the most informative indicators of innate and adaptive cellular immunity in diagnosing and monitoring SIRS-induced immunosuppression.

2. Neutrophils

Circulating numbers of neutrophils in blood are commonly increased by the rapid egress from the bone marrow and recruitment from the marginal pool to the circulating one.

Most studied have reported inconsistent alterations in the function of neutrophils in patients with sepsis at the early phase (impaired bacterial phagocytosis (activated or decreased, incomplete phagocytosis), increased synthesis of reactive oxygen species (ROS), decreased chemotaxis) [6]. Existing neutrophil dysfunction may be furtherly aggravated or reversed. Therefore, impaired neutrophil function preludes insufficient bacterial clearance and neutrophil dysfunction and increases the susceptibility to infection [7]. It is worth noting that patients with severe neutrophil dysfunction are more prone to nosocomial and secondary infections [8]. Flow cytometry allows evaluating cell functional properties, but the interaction of external and internal factors (disease staging, blood sampling technique, sample storage, and preparation) should be taken into account before interpreting the obtained results.

Neutrophils are well-known highly informative predictors of adverse complications in patients with sepsis. Immature neutrophils with decreased expression of CD10 and CD16 (CD10-/CD16low) have exhibited an immunosuppression pattern implying the presence of the link with increased early mortality in patients with sepsis [9]. A unique CD10-/CD16low immature neutrophil subpopulation has been studied in cardiac patients. An increase in their concentration has been recorded even in the perioperative period. Thus, CD10-/CD16low neutrophils represent a significant portion of the circulating pool after cardiac surgery (over 40% of circulating neutrophils), emerge a left shift, and influence the phenotype and functional activity of circulating neutrophils [10].

3. Monocytes and macrophages

Monocytes and macrophages play a pivotal role in triggering and regulating the immune responses [11]. Monocytes and macrophages are key players in the formation of the cytokine storm in the hyperactive phase of SIRS and sepsis. They are an important link with the onset and maintenance immunosuppression. Endotoxin tolerance is a well-known functional defect in monocytes and macrophages [12], displaying a decrease in the release of pro-inflammatory cytokines in response to endotoxin (LPS) and other types of TLR stimuli [12]. Endotoxin tolerance may be induced in circulating monocytes as well as reticular spleen monocytes (splenocytes). It is directly related to immunosuppression, since a decrease in cytokine production blocks further expansion of the immune responses and limits the involvement of the cells of the adaptive immune system.

There are two in vitro assays evaluating the ability of monocytes to respond to the provocation of the immune system and detecting induced immunosuppression. The first includes the measurement of cytokines in cell culture supernatant in response to stimulation [13], whereas the second one assesses intracellular synthesis of cytokines. Fumeaux et al. have measured the level of production of intracellular cytokines and reported that monocytes in septic patients possess predominant anti-inflammatory phenotype with an increase in the intracellular ratio of IL10/TNF [14].

Main mechanisms implicated in the induction of monocyte and macrophage endotoxin tolerance in septic and sterile SIRS are considered as universal. Hyporeactivity has been repeatedly reported in septic patients, whereas endotoxin tolerance exhibited by monocytes has been first described in patients undergoing aortic surgery or those suffering from thermal trauma, hepatic/renal ischemia-reperfusion injury, coronary occlusion, and hemorrhagic shock [15]. However, the protective mechanisms of immunosuppression at the initial phase of hyperactivation of the immune response in patients with SIRS and sepsis may aggravate and lead to adverse events. In addition to endotoxin tolerance, anergy of monocytes and macrophages may be induced [16], capable to transit the last to an immunosuppressive state with the impaired antigen-presenting ability [17] and increased risk of nosocomial infections and adverse complications. The immunosuppressive phenotype of monocytes in SIRS and sepsis is characterized by a decrease in the expression of key MHC II genes and co-stimulating molecules (CD86, CD40, and HLA-DR), mediating a violation of antigen-presenting ability.

In addition, patients with sepsis-induced immunosuppression, as well as after cardioplegia during cardiac surgery, have demonstrated a significant decrease in the expression of the chemokine receptor CX3CR1 (receptor for fractalkine). Since the CX3CR1/CX3CL1 interaction mediates chemotaxis, adhesion, and migration of pro-inflammatory cells to the damaged area or infection, leading to tissue infiltration [18], its decreased expression on monocytes may prevent their migration with further phagocytosis and lesion sanitation.

Decreased cell surface expression of major histocompatibility complex class II (MHC II) is a key marker of suppressive functional rearrangement of monocytes. Indeed, low HLA-DR expression on monocytes has reported the correlation with lower synthesis of TNF-a and IL-1 in response to stimulation [19], decreased antigen-presenting ability [20], and expression level of the CD86 co-stimulatory molecule [21]. This biomarker is commonly used to monitor immunosuppression in various critical conditions. Clinical studies have reported that the magnitude and overtime persistence of HLA-DR reduction on monocytes correlates with an increase in mortality and the incidence of infections [22] associated with medical care provision in ICU patients [23]. It is worth noting that the monitoring of HLA-DR expression on monocytes during the first days after surgery does not allow predicting an increased risk of postoperative SIRS or sepsis or infectious complications in patients undergoing cardiac surgery.

Functional tests have confirmed the presence of the suppressor phenotypic transit in monocytes and have demonstrated lower proliferation of T-lymphocytes in the LPS-stimulated mixed culture of lymphocytes and monocytes in septic patients than healthy donor monocytes.

4. Myeloid-derived suppressor cells (MDSC)

MDSCs are a heterogeneous population of immature myeloid cells with potent immunosuppressive activity against various types of cells, mainly T-lymphocytes. MDSCs have been first described in cancer patients as the cells capable to suppress the immune response, while orchestrating angiogenesis, invasion, and metastasis of tumors to the distant sites [24]. Certain difficulties have been experienced in comparing and interpreting data obtained in various research laboratories, caused mainly by the gap in the gating strategies and the description of the MDSC phenotype. In 2016, Bronte et al. published the recommendations for myeloid-derived suppressor cell nomenclature and characterization standards in 2016 and proposed to distinguish three main populations of MDSC: polymorphonuclear (PMN) or granulocytic MDSC (PMN-MDSC), monocytic MDSC (M-MDSC), and early-stage MDSC (eMDSC) [25].

The minimum set of the phenotypic criteria (but sufficient) to distinguish MDSC in humans is as follows:

M-MDSC: CD11b+CD14+HLA-DRlow/-CD15-
PMN-MDSC: – CD14-CD11b+CD15+ or CD11b+CD14–CD66b+
eMDSC: Lin– (including CD3, CD14, CD15, CD19, CD56) HLA-DR–CD33+

M-MDSCs suppress both antigen-specific and non-specific T-cell responses associated with the production of NO and cytokines. PMN-MDSCs are capable of suppressing antigen-specific immune responses. The secretion of reactive oxygen species (ROS) by M-MDSC and PMN-MDSC is an important mechanism associated with the induction of the antigen-specific immune T-cell tolerance [26].

An early increase in MDSCs is associated with early mortality, while their persistent expansion with the prolonged length of stay in the ICU. Multivariate analysis has proved that a persistent increase in PMN-MDSCs appeared to be a strong independent predictor of nosocomial infections and poor prognosis [27], indicating the transition of the septic process to the induced immunosuppression. However, this transition is defined not only for sepsis, but also for other systemic inflammatory responses. Elevated levels of PMN-MDSC in patients at admission to the ICU is a strong predictor of mortality in the first 7 days. An increase in arginase in these patients directly correlates with the level of PMN-MDSC [28]. Various studies have shown a decrease in plasma concentrations of arginine in critical patients [29] with immunosuppression.

5. Dendritic cells

Dendritic cells (DCs) are short-lived immune cells. Dendritic cell precursors originated from the bone marrow enter the bloodstream (circulating DCs) and then migrate to the tissues (tissue DCs), with most of the DCs being present in the tissues. DCs are antigen-presenting cells that induce T-cell immune responses, and the cytokines synthesized by DC activate innate and adaptive immunity [30].

Most of the studies are focused on the quantitative and qualitative assessment of DCs in patients with sepsis-induced immunosuppression, but few of them examines these processes in noninfectious SIRS. A decrease in the number of circulating DCs has been reported in patients with sepsis [31] and septic shock [32]. A significant decrease in the number of DC in spleens of septic patients who died has been found compared to trauma patients [33].

In systemic inflammatory response syndrome, DCs are well-known to be vulnerable to apoptosis. In addition, the induction of mDC and pDC apoptosis promotes prolonged immunosuppression and persistence of infection [34]. The change of phenotype is closely associated with a decrease in the number of DCs. Thus, SIRS- and sepsis-induced immunosuppression are accompanied by a decrease in the antigen-presenting ability of DCs leading to reduced expression of HLA-DR, co-stimulatory molecules CD80/86, and transcription factor IRF4. It is worth noting that anti-inflammatory properties are activated in DCs, including increased synthesis of IL-10 and TGFβ [6]. Thus, the number of circulating DCs and the expression of HLA-DR may be a promising biomarker of SIRS- and sepsis-induced immunosuppression that requires further studies, including the use of flow cytometry.

6. Lymphopenia

Lymphopenia results in decreased resistance to pathogenic microorganisms and is considered as a non-specific yet commonly used marker of immunosuppression in critically ill patients [35]. If the adaptive immune system is weakened, the body has difficulties properly coordinating the fight against the pathogen leading to persistent primary or secondary infections. Depletion of each subpopulation of lymphocytes occurs (with the exception of regulatory T cells, see below) in the immunosuppressive phase of the disease. The degree of lymphopenia correlates with the development of health-associated infections and/or mortality within 28 days [36]. It is important to note that protracted lymphopenia in ICU patients is associated with the presence of infectious complications [37], and this indicator is a better predictor of bacteremia than C-reactive protein and white blood cell count.

7. NK cells, γδ-lymphocytes, mucosal-associated invariant T-lymphocytes

Flow cytometry have reported a significant decrease in the number of circulating NK cells in patients with severe trauma and sepsis. A long-term decrease in NK cells correlates with an increase in mortality [38]. In addition, a decrease in cytotoxicity and antibody-dependent cytotoxicity of NK cells during sepsis have been previously reported [39].

Septic patients also have a decrease in circulating mucosal-associated invariant T-lymphocytes (MAIT) [40], while a persistent decrease in MAIT correlates with the subsequent development of health-associated infections.

A significant decrease in the relative content of **γ**δ-lymphocytes has been found in patients with sepsis with prevailing non-proliferating **γ**δ-lymphocyte population [41].

8. T-lymphocytes

8.1 Quantitative changes in T-lymphocytes

Quantitative and functional changes in T-lymphocytes occur in patients with induced immunosuppression. They include activation of apoptosis, anergy, and depletion, an increase in the percentage of Treg cells. Each of these changes will be considered separately.

One of the causes of lymphopenia in immunosuppression is associated with the death of T and B lymphocytes through apoptosis. There are a lot of evidences confirming a decrease in the number of circulating and deep depletion of tissue resident CD4 + and CD8 + T-lymphocytes during sepsis [42].

8.2 Programmed cell death receptor 1 (PD-1) and its ligand (PD-L1)

An important mechanism for enhancing apoptotic cell death is associated with increased expression of the programmed cell death receptor 1 (PD-1) and its ligand (PD-L1). PD-1 is a negative co-inhibitory molecule expressed by lymphocytes, myeloid cells, and DC. Under physiological conditions, PD-1 is associated with negative regulation of the immune system by preventing the activation of T-lymphocytes, which reduces autoimmunity and increases self-tolerance. The inhibitory effect of PD-1 is through stimulation of apoptosis of antigen-specific T-lymphocytes in the lymph nodes and a decrease in apoptosis of regulatory T-lymphocytes (Treg). The main PD-1 ligand (PD-L1) expresses epithelial cells, endothelial cells, and antigen-presenting cells (APCs) [43]. Flow cytometry reported that the expression of PD-1 on T-lymphocytes and PD-L1 on monocytes drastically increased in patients with septic shock and led to accelerated apoptosis of all major lymphocyte subpopulations compared to healthy volunteers [44]. Macrophages also express higher PD-1 levels during sepsis, which is associated with dysfunction of these cells and a decrease in microbial clearance [45].

Excess expression of PD-1 and PD-L1 on immune cells leads to their deactivation and acceleration of apoptotic death, resulting in the formation and development of sepsis- and SIRS-induced immunosuppression [46]. Day et al. have found an increase in the expression of PD-1 and PD-L1 on CD4 + T-lymphocytes within the first 5 days of hospitalization in patients with sepsis and severe trauma compared with healthy donors. The expression level of PD-1 and PD-L1 correlated with a decrease in stimulated proliferative lymphocyte activity and an increase in the concentration of IL-10 (anti-inflammatory cytokine) in the blood [47].

In addition to the direct apoptotic effects of PD-1 and PD-L1 molecules on T-lymphocytes, they indirectly affect the number of antigen-presenting DCs. Antigen-presenting cells (APC) activate CD4+ T-lymphocytes, which quickly proliferate (clonal expansion is a feature common to all adaptive immune responses) and differentiate into different effector lines, namely, Th1, Th2, and Th17. The decrease in the number of DCs suppresses clonal expansion along with the direct apoptotic effects of PD-1/PD-L1, which may lead to a pronounced decrease in the number of B- and T-lymphocytes [33].

Experimental and clinical trials have proved the pivotal role of PD-1 and PD-L1 in the pathogenesis of induced immunosuppression. The correlation of the expression of these molecules on the surfaces of immune cells with the development of infectious complications and an unfavorable outcome has been determined. Thus, a high level of PD-L1 expression on neutrophils correlates with an increase in the blood levels of pro- and anti-inflammatory cytokines and an unfavorable outcome in septic patients [48]. A relationship between the increased expression of PD-1 on monocytes in patients with septic shock and mortality and the risk of secondary nosocomial infections has been recently reported. Similarly, an increase in PD-1 and PD-L1 by Th also correlates with an increase in the number of secondary nosocomial infections and mortality after septic shock and severe trauma [49].

8.3 Qualitative changes in T-lymphocytes

In addition to a quantitative decrease in CD4 + T-lymphocytes, there is a simultaneous decrease in cytokine production and a decrease in the main transcription factors in the Th1 and Th2 populations (T-bet for Th1 cells, GATA3 for Th2 cells) in patients with sepsis [50]. These processes are associated with anergy and depletion of T-lymphocytes. The concept of depletion was introduced by Zajac to describe the impaired effector function of T cells [51]. Dysregulation of T-cell functions has been previously reported in patients with neonatal and pediatric sepsis and ICU patients with hemorrhagic shock and severe tissue damage followed by induced immunosuppression [52].

8.4 An increase in the relative number of Treg

T-lymphocyte dysfunction, if immunosuppression has induced, is associated with an increase in the relative number of circulating Treg lymphocytes subsets (T-cells with regulatory properties). Originally, this phenomenon was described in patients with septic shock [53]. Treg functions mainly at the site of inflammation, modulating the immune response via three main mechanisms: direct killing of cytotoxic cells, inhibition of cytokine production by cytotoxic cells, and direct secretion of immunomodulating anti-inflammatory cytokines, such as TGF-β and IL-10 [54]. An increase in Treg levels has been previously observed immediately after the shock but has persisted only in patients with unfavorable outcomes. One of the mechanisms includes Treg cells resistance to sepsis-induced apoptosis compared to other T-cell populations. Blood levels of Treg cells in ICU patients can be considered as a prognostic marker for the development of septic complications and adverse outcomes [55].

Thus, the relative number of Treg cells and the level of expression of CD39 on Treg cells require further detailed study that may provide novel insights into the diagnosis of SIRS- and sepsis-induced immunosuppression. However, accurate results of any multicenter study require standardization of Treg phenotyping approaches, since various staining protocols and gating strategies are used (CD4 + CD25 +, CD4 + CD25 + CD127-, CD4 + FOXP3 +, etc.).

8.5 B- and T-lymphocyte attenuator (BTLA) and cytotoxic T-lymphocyte antigen-4 (CTCTLA-4)

T-lymphocyte dysfunction can contribute to the induction of immunosuppression and subsequent mortality. BTLA and its ligand express a wide variety of cells, including T and B lymphocytes. BTLA is a co-inhibiting receptor that inhibits CD4 + T-cell and B-cell functions and also suppresses signaling in CD4 + T cells aimed at their survival. The relative number of BTLA +/CD4 + lymphocytes was significantly higher in septic patients than in non-septic ICU patients and was associated with the subsequent onset of secondary infections. CTLA-4, if interacting with CD80 or CD86, may be regarded as other inhibitory regulator in the early stages of T-cell activation and proliferation. CTLA-4 is an important inhibitor of the functional activity of immune cells, and its expression is increased in patients with sepsis [56].

9. Conclusion

The review proves that there are similar mechanisms underlying the induction of immunosuppression in septic and sterile systemic inflammatory processes and justifying the use of the term “injury-induced immunosuppression.” Immunological monitoring will allow distinguishing between the rapidly changing phases of progressive inflammation and severe immunosuppression to optimize early diagnosis and treatment (**Table 1**).

Marker	Status	Diagnostic significance or the underlying mechanism triggering immunosuppression	Prognostic value
% CD10-/CD16low out of the total concentration of neutrophils	↑	Immunosuppression	Sepsis-associated mortality
% CD62L dim out of the total concentration of neutrophils	↑	Immunosuppression	–
CD86 expression on monocytes	↓	Decrease in antigen-presenting function	Long-term decrease combined with a decrease in HLA-DR. Increased mortality and healthcare-associated infections
HLA-DR expression on monocytes or levels of M-MDSC	↓ ↑	Decrease in antigen-presenting function	Increased mortality and healthcare-associated infections
CX3CR1 expression on monocytes	↓	Reduction in monocyte chemotaxis	Increased mortality
PMN-MDSC	↑	T-cell-mediated suppression	Increased mortality and healthcare-associated infections
Blood levels of DCs	↓	Immunosuppression	Increased mortality and healthcare-associated infections
HLA-DR expression on DCs	↓	Decrease in antigen-presenting function	Increased mortality and healthcare-associated infections
Lymphopenia	↓	Immunosuppression	Increased mortality and healthcare-associated infections
PD1 expression on T-lymphocytes	↑	Enhanced apoptosis of T-lymphocytes	Increased mortality and healthcare-associated infections
PD-L1 expression on monocytes	↑	Enhanced apoptosis of all lymphocyte subpopulations	Increased mortality and healthcare-associated infections
Relative blood levels of Treg cells	↑	Immunosuppression	Increased mortality and healthcare-associated infections
CD39+ expression on Treg cells	↑	Immunosuppression	Differential diagnosis of sepsis and SIRS and increased mortality
BTLA and CTLA-4 expression on lymphocytes	↑	Suppression of lymphocyte activation and proliferation	–

Table 1.
Diagnostic and/or prognostic values of the main immunological parameters of flow cytometry associated with injury-induced immunosuppression in ICU patients.

Author details

Evgeny Grigoryev*, Vera Matveeva, Artem Ivkin and Maryam Khanova
Scientific Research Institute for Complex Issues of Cardiovascular Diseases, Kemerovo, Russian Federation

*Address all correspondence to: grigev@kemcardio.ru

References

[1] Medzhitov R, Schneider DS, Soares MP. Disease tolerance as a defense strategy. Science. 2012;**335**:936-941. DOI: 10.1126/science.1214935

[2] Hotchkiss RS, Monneret G, Payen D. Immunosuppression in sepsis: A novel understanding of the disorder and a new therapeutic approach. The Lancet Infectious Diseases. 2013;**13**:260-268. DOI: 10.1016/S1473-3099(13)70001-X

[3] Schefold JC, Hasper D, Reinke P, Monneret G, Volk HD. Consider delayed immunosuppression into the concept of sepsis. Critical Care Medicine. 2008;**36**(11):3118. DOI: 10.1097/CCM.0b013e31818bdd8f

[4] Ward NS, Casserly B, Ayala A. The compensatory anti-inflammatory response syndrome (CARS) in critically ill patients. Clinics in Chest Medicine. 2008;**29**(4):617-625. DOI: 10.1016/j.ccm.2008.06.010

[5] Monneret G, Venet F, Kullberg BJ, Netea MG. ICU-acquired immunosuppression and the risk for secondary fungal infections. Medical Mycology. 2011;**49**(Suppl 1):S17-S23. DOI: 10.3109/13693786.2010.509744

[6] Hotchkiss RS, Monneret G, Payen D. Sepsis-induced immunosuppression: From cellular dysfunctions to immunotherapy. Nature Reviews. Immunology. 2013;**13**:862-874. DOI: 10.1038/nri3552

[7] Delano MJ, Thayer T, Gabrilovich S, Kelly-Scumpia KM, Winfield RD, Scumpia PO, et al. Sepsis induces early alterations in innate immunity that impact mortality to secondary infection. Journal of Immunology. 2011;**186**:195-202. DOI: 10.4049/jimmunol.1002104

[8] Stephan F, Yang K, Tankovic J, Soussy CJ, Dhonneur G, Duvaldestin P, et al. Impairment of polymorphonuclear neutrophil functions precedes nosocomial infections in critically ill patients. Critical Care Medicine. 2002;**30**:315-322

[9] Marini O, Costa S, Bevilacqua D, Calzetti F, Tamassia N, Spina C, et al. Mature CD10+ and immature CD10− neutrophils present in G-CSF-treated donors display opposite effects on T cells. Blood. 2017;**129**(10):1343-1356. DOI: 10.1182/blood-2016-04-713206

[10] Orr Y, Taylor JM, Bannon PG, Geczy C, Kritharides L. Circulating CD10−/CD16 low neutrophils provide a quantitative index of active bone marrow neutrophil release. British Journal of Haematology. 2005;**131**(4):508-519. DOI: 10.1111/j.1365-2141.2005.05794.x

[11] Parihar A, Eubank TD, Doseff AI. Monocytes and macrophages regulate immunity through dynamic networks of survival and cell death. Journal of Innate Immunity. 2010;**2**:204-215. DOI: 10.1159/000296507

[12] Biswas SK, Lopez-Collazo E. Endotoxin tolerance: New mechanisms, molecules and clinical significance. Trends in Immunology. 2009;**30**:475-487. DOI: 10.1016/j.it.2009.07.009

[13] Fumeaux T, Dufour J, Stern S, Pugin J. Immune monitoring of patients with septic shock by measurement of intraleukocyte cytokines. Intensive Care Medicine. 2004;**30**:2028-2037. DOI: 10.1007/s00134-004-2429-8

[14] Cavaillon JM, Adrie C, Fitting C, Adib-Conquy M. Endotoxin tolerance: Is there a clinical relevance? Journal of Endotoxin Research. 2003;**9**(2):101-107. DOI: 10.1179/096805103125001487

[15] Lukaszewicz AC, Grienay M, Resche-Rigon M, Pirracchio R, Faivre V, Boval B, et al. Monocytic HLA-DR

expression in intensive care patients: Interest for prognosis and secondary infection prediction. Critical Care Medicine. 2009;**37**:2746-2752. DOI: 10.1097/CCM.0b013e3181ab858a

[16] Delano MJ, Ward PA. Sepsis-induced immune dysfunction: Can immune therapies reduce mortality? The Journal of Clinical Investigation. 2016;**126**:23-31. DOI: 10.1172/JCI82224

[17] Pachot A, Cazalis MA, Venet F, Turrel F, Faudot C, Voirin N, et al. Decreased expression of the fractalkine receptor CX3CR1 on circulating monocytes as new feature of sepsis-induced immunosuppression. Journal of Immunology. 2008;**180**:6421-6429. DOI: 10.4049/jimmunol.180.9.6421

[18] Piani A, Hossle JP, Birchler T, Siegrist CA, Heumann D, Davies G, et al. Expression of MHC class II molecules contributes to lipopolysaccharide responsiveness. European Journal of Immunology. 2000;**30**:3140-3146. DOI: 10.1002/1521-4141(200011)30:11<3140::AID-IMMU3140>3.0.CO;2-O

[19] Wolk K, Docke WD, von Baehr V, Volk HD, Sabat R. Impaired antigen presentation by human monocytes during endotoxin tolerance. Blood. 2000;**96**:218-223

[20] Wolk K, Höflich C, Zuckermann-Becker H, Döcke WD, Volk HD, Sabat R. Reduced monocyte CD86 expression in postinflammatory immunodeficiency. Critical Care Medicine. 2007;**35**(2):458-467. DOI: 10.1097/01.CCM.0000254724.54515.2F

[21] Venet F, Lukaszewicz AC, Payen D, Hotchkiss R, Monneret G. Monitoring the immune response in sepsis: A rational approach to administration of immunoadjuvant therapies. Current Opinion in Immunology. 2013;**25**:477-483. DOI: 10.1016/j.coi.2013.05.006

[22] Chenouard A, Braudeau C, Cottron N, Bourgoin P, Salabert N, Roquilly A, et al. HLA-DR expression in neonates after cardiac surgery under cardiopulmonary bypass: A pilot study. Intensive Care Medicine Experimental. 2018;**6**(1):1. DOI: 10.1186/s40635-017-0166-x

[23] Fabienne V, Cour M, Demaret J, Guillaume M, Laurent A. Decreased monocyte HLA-DR expression in patients after non-shockable out-of-hospital cardiac arrest. Shock. 2016;**46**(1):33-36. DOI: 10.1097/SHK.0000000000000561

[24] Umansky V, Sevko A. Tumor microenvironment and myeloid-derived suppressor cells. Cancer Microenvironment. 2013;**6**:169-177. DOI: 10.1007/s12307-012-0126-7

[25] Bronte V, Brandau S, Chen S-H, Colombo MP, Frey AB, Greten TF, et al. Recommendations for myeloid-derived suppressor cell nomenclature and characterization standards. Nature Communications. 2016;**7**:12150. DOI: 10.1038/ncomms12150

[26] Koehn BH, Apostolova P, Haverkamp JM, Miller JS, McCullar V, Tolar J, et al. GVHD-associated, inflammasome-mediated loss of function in adoptively transferred myeloid-derived suppressor cells. Blood. 2015;**126**:1621-1628. DOI: 10.1182/blood-2015-03-634691

[27] Uhel F, Azzaoui I, Grégoire M, Pangault C, Dulong J, Tadié JM, et al. Early expansion of circulating granulocytic myeloid-derived suppressor cells predicts development of nosocomial infections in septic patients. American Journal of Respiratory and Critical Care Medicine. 2017;**196**(3):315-327. DOI: 10.1164/rccm.201606-1143OC

[28] Gey A, Tadie JM, Caumont-Prim A, Hauw-Berlemont C, Cynober L, Fagon JY, et al. Granulocytic

myeloid-derived suppressor cells inversely correlate with plasma arginine and overall survival in critically ill patients. Clinical and Experimental Immunology. 2015;**180**(2):280-288. DOI: 10.1111/cei.12567

[29] Tadié JM, Cynober L, Peigne V, Caumont-Prim A, Neveux N, Gey A, et al. Arginine administration to critically ill patients with a low nitric oxide fraction in the airways: A pilot study. Intensive Care Medicine. 2013;**39**(9):1663-1665. DOI: 10.1007/s00134-013-2984-y

[30] Steinman RM, Hemmi H. Dendritic cells: Translating innate to adaptive immunity. Current Topics in Microbiology and Immunology. 2006;**311**:17-58

[31] Riccardi F, Della Porta MG, Rovati B, Casazza A, Radolovich D, De Amici M, et al. Flow cytometric analysis of peripheral blood dendritic cells in patients with severe sepsis. Cytometry. Part B, Clinical Cytometry. 2011;**80**:14-21. DOI: 10.1002/cyto.b.20540

[32] Guisset O, Dilhuydy MS, Thiebaut R, Lefevre J, Camou F, Sarrat A, et al. Decrease in circulating dendritic cells predicts fatal outcome in septic shock. Intensive Care Medicine. 2007;**33**:148-152. DOI: 10.1007/s00134-006-0436-7

[33] Hotchkiss RS, Tinsley KW, Swanson PE, Grayson MH, Osborne DF, Wagner TH, et al. Depletion of dendritic cells, but not macrophages, in patients with sepsis. Journal of Immunology. 2002;**168**:2493-2500. DOI: 10.4049/jimmunol.168.5.2493

[34] Pastille E, Didovic S, Brauckmann D, Rani M, Agrawal H, Schade FU, et al. Modulation of dendritic cell differentiation in the bone marrow mediates sustained immunosuppression after polymicrobial sepsis. Journal of Immunology. 2011;**186**:977-986. DOI: 10.4049/jimmunol.1001147

[35] Adrie C, Lugosi M, Sonneville R, Souweine B, Ruckly S, Cartier JC, et al. Persistent lymphopenia is a risk factor for ICU-acquired infections and for death in ICU patients with sustained hypotension at admission. Shock. 2014;**42**:383-391. DOI: 10.1186/s13613-017-0242-0

[36] Inoue S, Suzuki-Utsunomiya K, Okada Y, Taira T, Iida Y, Miura N, et al. Reduction of immunocompetent T cells followed by prolonged lymphopenia in severe sepsis in the elderly. Critical Care Medicine. 2013;**41**:810-819. DOI: 10.1097/CCM.0b013e318274645f

[37] De Jager CPC, van Wijk PTL, Mathoera RB, de Jongh-Leuvenink J, van der Poll T, Wever PC. Lymphocytopenia and neutrophil-lymphocyte count ratio predict bacteremia better than conventional infection markers in an emergency care unit. Critical Care. 2010;**14**(5):R192. DOI: 10.1186/cc9309

[38] Forel J-M, Chiche L, Thomas G, Mancini J, Farnarier C, Cognet C, et al. Phenotype and functions of natural killer cells in critically-ill septic patients. PLoS One. 2012;7:e50446. DOI: 10.1186/cc9309

[39] Souza-Fonseca-Guimaraes F, Parlato M, Fitting C, Cavaillon JM, Adib-Conquy M. NK cell tolerance to TLR agonists mediated by regulatory T cells after polymicrobial sepsis. Journal of Immunology. 2012;**188**:5850-5858. DOI: 10.4049/jimmunol.1103616

[40] Grimaldi D, Le Bourhis L, Sauneuf B, Dechartres A, Rousseau C, Ouaaz F, et al. Specific MAIT cell behaviour among innate-like T lymphocytes in critically ill patients with severe infections. Intensive Care Medicine. 2014;**40**(2):192-201. DOI: 10.1007/s00134-013-3163-x

[41] Venet F, Bohe J, Debard AL, Bienvenu J, Lepape A, Monneret G. Both percentage of gammadelta T lymphocytes and CD3 expression are reduced during septic shock. Critical Care Medicine. 2005;**33**:2836-2840. DOI: 10.1097/01.CCM.0000189745.66585.AE

[42] Hotchkiss RS, Nicholson DW. Apoptosis and caspases regulate death and inflammation in sepsis. Nature Reviews. Immunology. 2006;**6**:813-822. DOI: 10.1038/nri1943

[43] Chen L, Flies DB. Molecular mechanisms of T cell co-stimulation and co-inhibition. Nature Reviews. Immunology. 2013;**13**(4):227-242. DOI: 10.1038/nri3405

[44] Zhang Y, Li J, Lou J, Zhou Y, Bo L, Zhu J, et al. Upregulation of programmed death-1 on T cells and programmed death ligand-1 on monocytes in septic shock patients. Critical Care. 2011;**15**(1):R70. DOI: 10.1186/cc10059

[45] Huang X, Venet F, Wang YL, Lepape A, Yuan Z, Chen Y, et al. PD-1 expression by macrophages plays a pathologic role in altering microbial clearance and the innate inflammatory response to sepsis. Proceedings of the National Academy of Sciences of the United States of America. 2009;**106**(15):6303-6308. DOI: 10.1073/pnas.0809422106

[46] Guignant C, Lepape A, Huang X, Kherouf H, Denis L, Poitevin F, et al. Programmed death-1 levels correlate with increased mortality, nosocomial infection and immune dysfunctions in septic shock patients. Critical Care. 2011;**15**:R99. DOI: 10.1186/cc10112

[47] Day CL, Kaufmann DE, Kiepiela P, Brown JA, Moodley ES, Reddy S, et al. PD-1 expression on HIV-specific T cells is associated with T-cell exhaustion and disease progression. Nature. 2006;**443**:350-354. DOI: 10.1038/nature05115

[48] Huang X, Chen Y, Chung CS, Yuan Z, Monaghan SF, Wang F, et al. Identification of B7-H1 as a novel mediator of the innate immune/proinflammatory response as well as a possible myeloid cell prognostic biomarker in sepsis. Journal of Immunology. 2014;**192**(3):1091-1099. DOI: 10.4049/jimmunol.1302252

[49] Goyert SM, Silver J. Editorial: PD-1, a new target for sepsis treatment: Better late than never. Journal of Leukocyte Biology. 2010;**88**:225-226. DOI: 10.1189/jlb.0410240

[50] Wick M, Kollig E, Muhr G, Koller M. The potential pattern of circulating lymphocytes TH1/TH2 is not altered after multiple injuries. Archives of Surgery. 2000;**135**:1309-1314. DOI: 10.1001/archsurg.135.11.1309

[51] Zajac AJ, Blattman JN, Murali-Krishna K, Sourdive DJD, Suresh M, Altman JD, et al. Viral immune evasion due to persistence of activated T cells without effector function. The Journal of Experimental Medicine. 1998;**188**:2205-2213. DOI: 10.1084/jem.188.12.2205

[52] Kuethe JW, Mintz-Cole R, Johnson BL 3rd, Midura EF, Caldwell CC, Schneider BS. Assessing the immune status of critically ill trauma patients by flow cytometry. Nursing Research. 2014;**63**(6):426-434. DOI: 10.1097/NNR.0000000000000061

[53] Monneret G, Debard AL, Venet F, Bohe J, Hequet O, Bienvenu J, et al. Marked elevation of human circulating CD41CD251 regulatory T cells in sepsis-induced immunoparalysis. Critical Care Medicine. 2003;**31**:2068-2071. DOI: 10.1097/01.CCM.0000069345.78884.0F

[54] Kessel A, Bamberger E, Masalha M, Toubi E. The role of T regulatory cells in

human sepsis. Journal of Autoimmunity. 2009;**32**(3-4):211-215. DOI: 10.1016/j.jaut.2009.02.014

[55] Chen K, Zhou QX, Shan HW, Li WF, Lin ZF. Prognostic value of CD4(1) CD25(1) Tregs as a valuable biomarker for patients with sepsis in ICU. World Journal of Emergency Medicine. 2015;**6**:40-43. DOI: 10.5847/wjem.j.1920-8642.2015.01.007

[56] Huang H, Xu R, Lin F, Bao C, Wang S, Ji C, et al. High circulating CD39(+) regulatory T cells predict poor survival for sepsis patients. International Journal of Infectious Diseases. 2015;**30**:57-63. DOI: 10.1016/j.ijid.2014.11.006

Chapter 2

Biological Modulation of the Treg: Teff Ratio: From Immunosuppression to Immunoactivation

Xining Yang and Mark D. Scott

Abstract

T cell-mediated immunomodulation can be, in simple terms, defined as altering the normal Treg:Teff ratio. Immunosuppression skews the net Treg:Teff ratio toward the 'tolerogenic' Treg component, while immunoactivation skews the response toward the 'proinflammatory' Teff component. In the treatment of autoimmune diseases, achieving an immunosuppressive state is a desirable goal in order to prevent ongoing injury by activated Teff cells. In contrast, an innate, or induced, immunosuppressive state can be deleterious and prevent pathogen-induced disease while allow for the progression of cancer. Indeed, a current goal of cancer therapy is attenuating an existing endogenous immunosuppressive state that prevents effective T cell-mediated immunorecognition of cancer cells. Thus, the biological modulation of the Treg:Teff ratio provides a unique approach for treating both autoimmune diseases and cancers. Using a biomanufacturing system, miRNA-enriched immunotherapeutic has been generated that either induce (TA1) or overcome (IA1) an immunosuppressive state. As will be shown, these therapeutics show efficacy both in vitro and in vivo in the prevention of autoimmune Type 1 diabetes and in enhancing the ability of resting immune cells to recognize and inhibit cancer cell growth. The successful development of these cost-effective, and easily biomanufactured, secretome-based therapeutics may prove useful in treating both autoimmune diseases and cancer.

Keywords: T lymphocyte, immunosuppression, immunoactivation, Treg, Teff, proinflammatory, autoimmunity, cancer, biomanufacturing, miRNA

1. Introduction

The core function of the immune system is preserving *'self'* and rejecting 'non-self'. Biologically, 'non-self' is most often seen as exogenous biologicals (e.g., viruses and bacteria), abnormal autologous cells (e.g., cancers) and, more recently, 'man-made diseases' arising from the purposeful introduction of *'non-self'* (e.g., enzyme-replacement therapy, transfusion and transplantation medicine). Immunological *'self'* of most tissues is imparted by the major histocompatibility complex (MHC) which encodes a variety of proteins that provide a means for identifying, targeting, and eliminating foreign invaders and diseased cells while preserving normal *'self'* tissue [1–3]. The MHC proteins themselves consist of three classes. MHC Class I molecules are expressed on virtually all nucleated cells while Class II molecules are expressed exclusively on antigen presenting cells (APC; e.g., monocytes, macrophages, dendritic cell, B lymphocytes, and endothelial cells) and activated T lymphocytes. MHC Class III genes encode components of the complement system. The human MHC is referred to as the Human Leukocyte Antigen (HLA) complex while the murine equivalent is referred to as the Histocompatibility-2 (H2) complex. In the context of MHC-mediated immune recognition, the T lymphocyte (T cell) is of particular importance and plays a (the) central role in transfusion-associated graft versus host disease, transplant rejection, autoimmune diseases and cancer therapy. In terms of human diseases, autoimmune disorders and cancer are of most significance clinically.

The activation status of T cells plays a critical role in normal immunological homeostasis, the response to cancers, rejection of tissue/organ grafts, and the ontogeny and pathophysiology of autoimmune diseases. T cells encompass multiple subpopulations that can exert either a protolerogenic effects (regulatory T cells; Tregs) or a proinflammatory responses (effector T cells; Teff). Hence, in examining the immune status, the relative abundance of Tregs and Teff, i.e., the Treg:Teff ratio, is critical. Indeed, skewing the immune response towards either end of the continuum leads to significant medical consequences. As shown in **Figure 1**, an immunosuppressive state (increased Treg and/or decreased Teff) may facilitate the growth and spread of abnormal (i.e., cancer) cells, or in the context of transplantation medicine enhance engraftment, while a proinflammatory state (decreased Tregs and/or increased Teff) that may give rise to an autoimmune disease, graft rejection or, in the case of cancer, enhance tumor cell elimination. Indeed, modern clinical approaches attempt to pharmacologically modulate the Treg:Teff ratio in the treatment of autoimmune disease, tissue transplantation and cancer therapy.

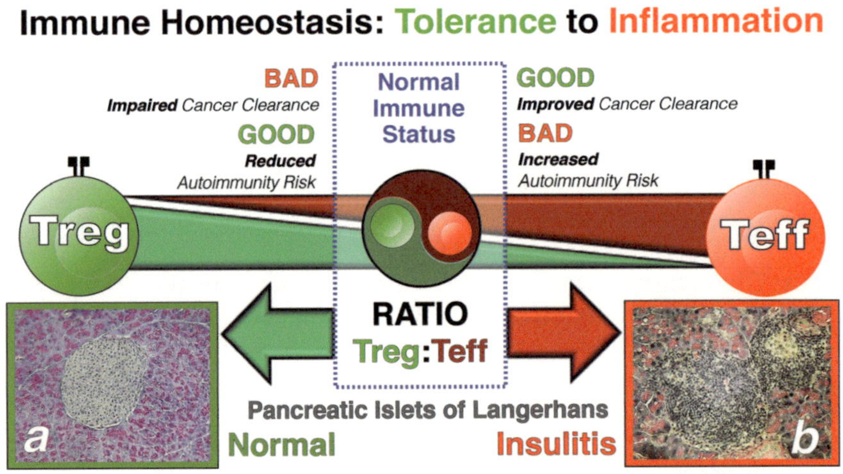

Figure 1.
The yin and yang of the cellular immune response. A key aspect of immune regulation is the dualism of the tolerogenic (Treg; e.g., Foxp3$^+$, IL-10$^+$, TGF-β$^+$ and IL-4$^+$) and effector (Teff; e.g., Th17$^+$, IL-2$^+$, INF-γ$^+$ IL-12$^+$, and TNF-β$^+$) CD4$^+$ T cells. Effector T cells also include cytotoxic CD8$^+$ T cells (CTL). These seemingly disparate cellular subpopulations are actually complementary, interconnected, and interdependent in regulating the immunological response. As such, the immune response is a continuum that may be best reflected by the Treg:Teff ratio. Indeed, the skewing of the Treg:Teff ratio towards either the left or right influences the immunological risks/benefits of an animal. As shown, a skewed response towards the Treg cells may prevent T1D or could be used to prevent rejection of transplanted islets. In contrast, skewing towards the Teff populations increases the risk of autoimmune diseases such as type 1 diabetes (T1D) consequent to the development of insulitis of the islet cells.

2. Autoimmune diseases: increasing the Treg:Teff ratio

Autoimmune diseases affect virtually all tissues and organs and encompass such diverse diseases as Type 1 Diabetes (T1D), Crohn's disease (CD), Multiple Sclerosis (MS), Rheumatoid Arthritis (RA) and immune thrombocytopenia (ITP). Despite the diversity of tissues affected, extensive research has demonstrated the central role for T cells with Treg being downregulated and Teff upregulated leading to a reduced Treg:Teff ratio and a chronic pro-inflammatory state (**Figure 1**). Current clinical approaches to regulating the Treg:Teff ratio are almost entirely focused on reducing the Teff component. Most commonly, treatments for chronic autoimmune diseases include administration of systemic steroids (e.g., dexamethasone), cytotoxic anti-proliferative/activation agents (e.g., cyclosporine), and interruption of proinflammatory cytokine signaling cascades (e.g., Enbrel) resulting in the induction of a general immunosuppressive state in the individual (**Figure 2**). While these pharmacological approaches are often highly effective in controlling the autoimmune disease, they also pose significant risks to the individual including increased risks of opportunistic infections, cancer and organ injury. Perhaps surprisingly, very few clinical tools exist to increase the Treg component of the Treg:Teff ratio. Importantly, an increase in the functional Treg component would be very effective at reducing the damage induced by the Teff subsets in autoimmune diseases and decreasing the risk of Host versus graft disease in tissue/organ transplantation.

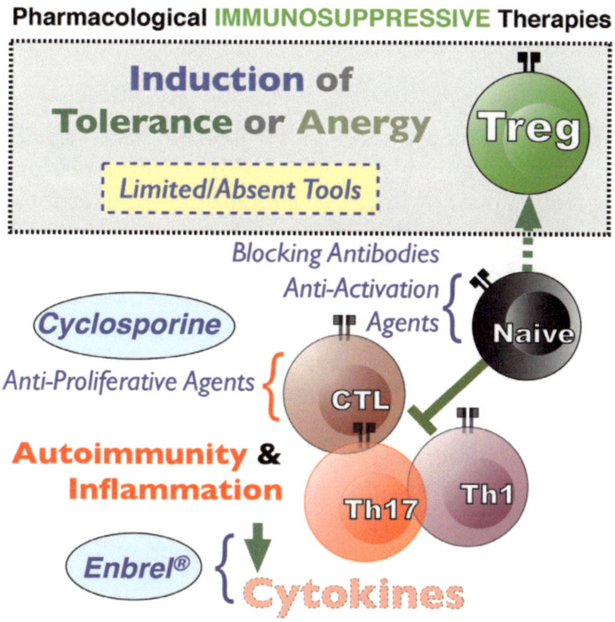

Figure 2.
Current pharmacologic therapies almost exclusively targets T cell activation and the Teff subpopulations. The proliferation of pro-inflammatory T cells (e.g., CTL, Th17, Th1 populations) and decrease in regulatory T cells (Treg) are commonly observed in both autoimmune and allorecognition immune responses. The majority of current therapeutic agents are primarily cytotoxic agents preventing T cell activation (e.g., cyclosporine and rapamycin) or T cell proliferation (e.g., methotrexate, corticosteroids and azathioprine). Additionally, some blocking antibodies have been investigated. In contrast, very limited, if any, pharmaceutical approaches are effective at increasing the Treg populations.

3. Cancer immunotherapy: decreasing the Treg:Teff ratio

In contrast to autoimmune diseases, immunosuppressive states (i.e., increased Treg:Teff ratio) exist resulting in a failure to appropriately respond to abnormal

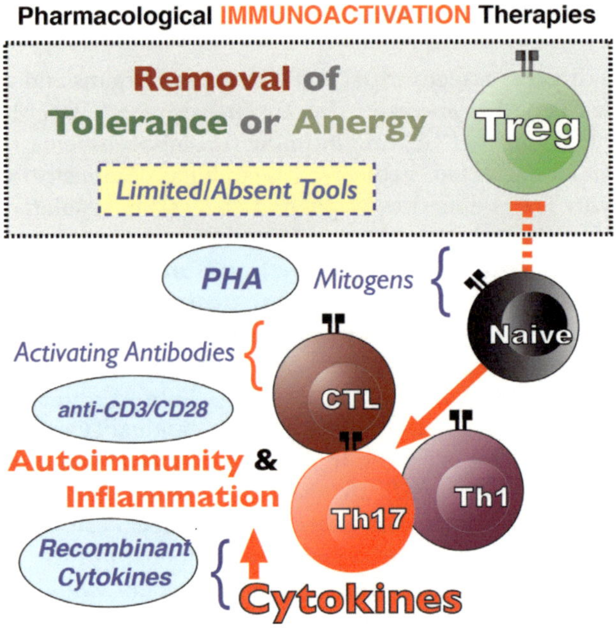

Figure 3.
Pharmacologic immunoactivation approaches have proven problematic due to their induction of poorly controlled inflammatory responses. A common cause of toxicity to these approaches has been the induction of the cytokine release syndrome (i.e., cytokine storm) [4–6].

cells (e.g., cancer) or infective agents (e.g., viruses and bacteria). This immunosuppressive state is most commonly exemplified by the progression and metastases of cancers arising from a poor or impaired cellular immune response to abnormal cells. Indeed, cancer progression is most often characterized by an impaired Teff response; either due to failure in recognizing abnormal cells (i.e., *'non-self'*) or via an existing immunosuppressive state arising from pharmacological agents or an inherent skewing of the Treg:Teff response towards the Treg cells. Unlike immunosuppressive diseases, the focus of clinical therapy has historically focused on cytotoxic chemicals that exert an enhanced lethality to cancer cells; though it is crucial to note that these agents also exhibit toxicity to normal cells, especially populations characterized by high proliferation rates (e.g., bone marrow; intestinal epithelial cells). Only more recently has cancer therapy began to focus on immunomodulation; in essence actively modulating the Treg:Teff ratio. Cancer immunotherapy has most commonly utilized cytokine therapy or direct activation of T cells via mitogens or monoclonal antibody therapy (**Figure 3**). However, both of these approaches are beset by systemic toxicity limiting their practical use. More recently, adoptive cellular therapeutic (ACT) approaches, using either allogenic T cells and/or CAR-T cells, have been used. However, while clearly an increasingly important cancer immunotherapy, these cellular approaches are expensive and, to date, continue to pose a risk of uncontrolled immune activation and bystander cell injury [4–6].

4. Biological modulation of the immune response

While pharmacologic agents remain the mainstay of modern medicine in treating both autoimmune diseases and cancers, a more direct ability to biologically modulate the Treg:Teff ratio could, potentially, be a safer and more effective tool in treating disease. It is worth noting that the biological modulation of the immune response is not a new concept. Indeed, the theory and practice of proinflammatory (*i.e.,* decreasing the Treg:Teff ratio) immunotherapy originated with William Coley's treatment in 1891 of cancer patients with bacteria (and other toxins) in order to induce an immune response that would exert a bystander effect on the tumor mass [7–10]. This pioneering clinical research has led to the recognition of Coley as the *"Father of Immunotherapy"*. Indeed, *Coley's Toxins* were a mainstay of cancer therapy for much of the early twentieth century and were marketed up to ~1962. However, these biologics were poorly defined, subject to diverse manufacturing standards (or lack thereof), and highly variable in their efficacy. By the mid twentieth century, criticisms from within the medical community led to less usage of *Coley's Toxins* as they were supplanted by the newer, and *'safer'*, developments of radiation therapy and chemotherapy; ironically both of which are now recognized to pose very significant short- and long-term risks to the patient. Indeed, it is these risks that are today driving forces in rediscovering immunotherapy.

Today, ~130 years after *Coley's Toxins* made their initial debut, modern immunotherapy has begun to revisit Coley's core principles of modulating (i.e., inducing) the endogenous immune response. Several approaches have been pursued to enhance the patient's own immune response. Ironically, similarly to Coley's use of *Streptococcus pyogenes* and *Serratia marcescens*, genetically modified strains of *Salmonella sp.* as well as recombinant polioviruses have been used in tumor therapy to induce an inflammatory microenvironment at the tumor site [11–14]. Tumor-specific immunotherapy has also been explored in which cancer cells from patients have been isolated, irradiated and modified for the re-infusion into the patient in an attempt to enhance anti-tumor immune activation and improve tumor killing [15–19]. But perhaps the favored approach has been the application of adoptive cell transfer (ACT) immunotherapy and, especially, chimeric antigen receptor (CAR)-T cell therapy [20–22]. While CAR-T cells will prove to be a crucial tool in cancer immunotherapy, they are beset by significant issues including cost, manufacturing time (weeks-months) and the risk of inducing cytokine release syndrome [4–6].

However, of significant clinical importance, few studies/approaches to date have elucidated effective biological immunotherapeutic approaches for modulating the Treg:Teff ratio (**Figures 2** and **3**). The ability to biologically manipulate the Treg: Teff ratio in a controllable manner would be of significant benefit in the treatment of cancer as well as the treatment of autoimmune diseases and the prevention of graft rejection.

5. A new approach to the biomodulation of the Treg:Teff ratio

As described in the preceding sections, pharmacologic agents, the current mainstay of clinical medicine, are, relatively speaking, non-specific agents beset with often significant adverse side effects. Hence, over the last decade increasing research has been done on biologically modifying the innate Treg:Teff immune response. In this chapter we will discuss a novel biomodulatory approach that more effectively, and directly, target the Treg:Teff ratio by increasing or decreasing Treg cells while simultaneously, and inversely, decreasing of increasing Teff subsets (**Figure 4**). This approach, derived from our work on the polymer-based bioengineering of allogeneic T cells and their use directly, or via the production of acellular microRNA (miRNA), to induce a tolerogenic or proinflammatory state characterized by significant changes in the Treg:Teff ratio [23–35].

Biomanufacturing of these immunomodulatory therapeutics was accomplished using a rapid and inexpensive leukocyte allorecognition-based system (**Figure 4**) [34, 35]. The core component of the biomanufacturing system is, in essence, a two-way mixed lymphocyte reaction (MLR) in which MHC-disparate leukocyte populations (either human PBMC or murine splenocytes) are co-incubated. Previous work from our laboratory demonstrated that the covalent grafting (PEGylation) of methoxy(polyethylene glycol) [mPEG] to one leukocyte population resulted in abrogation of the MHC-mediated proliferation of Teff cells [23–42]. Moreover, these studies demonstrated that, consequent to impaired cell:cell communication (**Figure 4C**), the weak allostimulation induced a tolerogenic/anergic state both in vitro and in vivo (**Figure 4A**) [29–34, 41]. The PEGylated cells themselves, or the resultant purified Treg cells, can be adoptively transferred to induce systemic tolerance in the recipient. Importantly, our studies demonstrated that the secretome of PEGylated-MLR also exerted a tolerogenic effect in vitro and in vivo [25–27, 29–34]. In parallel to the PEGylated cells, the control MLR (**Figure 4B**) was used to

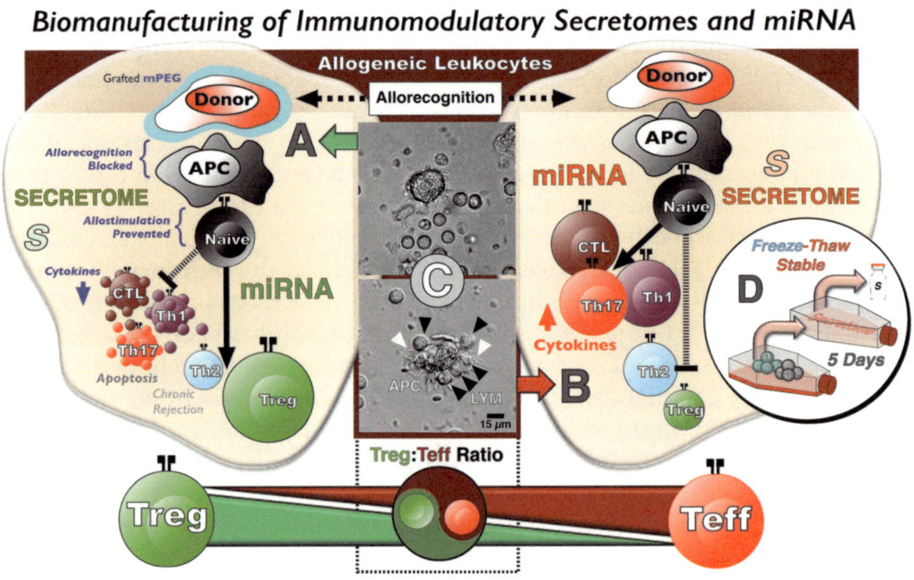

Figure 4.
Biomanufacturing immunomodulatory secretomes and purified miRNA. Panel A: Immunocamouflage of donor cells by the covalent grafting of methoxy(polyethylene) glycol (mPEG) to one donor population in a mixed lymphocyte reaction (MLR) results in the disruption of the essential cell–cell interactions (blue test) decreasing T cell proliferation and altered subset differentiation patterns. As shown, Treg cells are vastly increased while Teff subsets (CTL, Th1 and Th17 shown) are decreased resulting in an increase in the Treg:Teff ratio. Importantly, the secretome from the mPEG-MLR exerts a tolerogenic response when used either in vitro or in vivo. The key component of the secretome are miRNA. Panel B: Current pharmacologic therapy almost exclusively targets T cell activation and proliferation consequent to allorecognition. Response to non-self is in large part mediated by cell–cell interactions between antigen presenting cells (APC; e.g., dendritic cells) and naive T cells. This cell–cell interaction is characterized by essential adhesion, allorecognition and co-stimulation events. Consequent to allorecognition, a proliferation of proinflammatory T cells (e.g., cytotoxic T lymphocyte, CTL; Th17, IL-17^{+}*; Th1, IFN-γ*$^{+}$*; and IL-2*$^{+}$* populations) and decrease in regulatory T cells (Treg, Foxp3*$^{+}$* and CD25*$^{+}$*) is observed. Panel C: As shown in photomicrographs, in a control MLR, significant and persistent interactions (black arrows) occur between allogeneic lymphocytes (LYM) and dendritic cells (APC). The lymphocyte adhesion and antigen presentation interactions typically occur at pseudopodal extensions from the APC (white arrows). PEGylation of either allogeneic PBMC population decreases the stability and duration of initial cell:cell interactions between lymphocytes due to the global charge and steric camouflage of membrane proteins. Panel D: Importantly, the secretomes/miRNA bioproduction is both simple and rapid. As shown, allogeneic leukocytes (a, b) are incubated for 5 days and the secretome is collected. The secretome itself can be used or the miRNA component of the secretome can be further isolated for use. Both the secretome and miRNA can be stored frozen as they are stable under freeze–thaw conditions. The key component of the secretome are soluble (free and exosome) miRNA. Size of the T cell populations denotes increase or decrease in number. Apoptosis is indicated by blebbing. Data derived from Refs. [23–35]. Figure modified from Scott et al. [35].*

generate a proinflammatory secretome, or with further purification, miRNA preparation that could induce a controlled inflammatory response in unactivated T cells [25–27, 29–34]. Most importantly, the process is rapid (5 days), inexpensive and can be accomplished using stand tissue culture facilities—though also suitable for larger scale bioreactor systems (**Figure 4D**).

The two biomanufactured miRNA-enrich therapeutics, denoted as TA1 for the tolerogenic preparation and IA1 for the proinflammatory preparation, exert potent immunomodulatory effects on T cells differentiation (**Figure 5**). TA1 drives the differentiation of $CD3^{+}CD4^{-}CD8^{-}$ T cells towards Treg cells ($CD4^{+}Foxp3^{+}CD25^{+}$) while IA1 drives T cell proliferation towards both $CD4^{+}$ Th17 and Th1 cells and also towards $CD3^{+}CD8^{+}$ cytotoxic T lymphocytes (CTL). Thus, stable and storable (freeze–thaw stable) tolerogenic and proinflammatory biologics can be rapidly (5 days) and reproducibly biomanufactured.

Importantly, the active component of the TA1 and IA1 therapeutics are miRNAs—not cytokines or other potential immunomodulatory effectors [31, 34, 35]. The role of miRNA can be seen by the loss of immunomodulatory activity of TA1 and IA1 conditioned murine plasma upon treatment with RNase (**Figure 6**). As shown, naïve control mice (N) have high levels of Treg cells relative to Th17 cell. However, when challenged with a transfusion of allogeneic cells (AC), by day 5 Treg cells have decreased significantly with a concomitant increase in Th17. However, if naïve mice are pretreated with TA1 or IA1, the immune response to the allogeneic cells is dramatically altered. TA1 pre-treatment resulted in a maintenance, and slight elevation, of normal murine Treg levels and prevention of the Th17 upregulation upon allogeneic challenge. In contrast, IA1 pre-treatment enhanced the inflammatory response to the allogenic cells; i.e., significantly decreased Treg and increased Th17 cells relative to both naïve mice and control AC challenged mice. Importantly, RNase treatment of the TA1 or IA1 samples to degrade the miRNA component resulted in the attenuation of their respective immunomodulatory activity resulting in a T cell response virtually identical to the AC treated control mice.

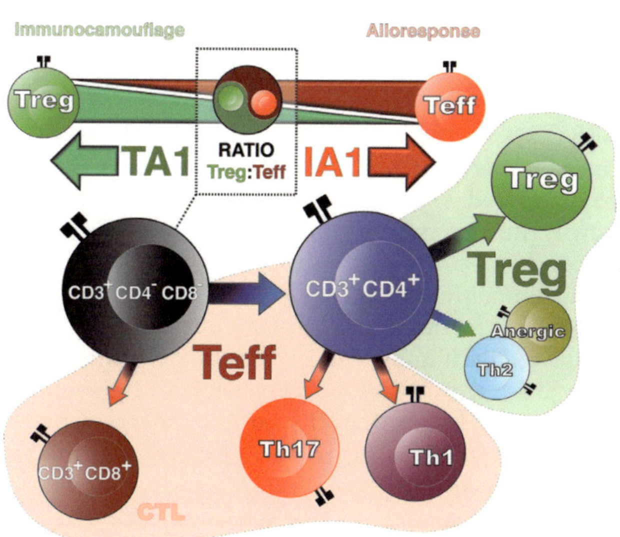

Figure 5.
In vitro and in vivo flow cytometric and functional analyses of T cells demonstrates that the TA1 and IA1 therapeutics differentially skew the differentiation pattern of naive $CD3^{+}CD4^{-}CD8^{-}$ T cells. As shown diagrammatically, TA1 favors tolerogenic/anergic T cell subsets while significantly inhibiting proinflammatory Teff populations. Conversely, as shown by the skewing of the Treg:Teff ratio, IA1 induces differentiation and proliferation of both $CD4^{+}$ and $CD8^{+}$ Teff subsets while reducing Treg populations.

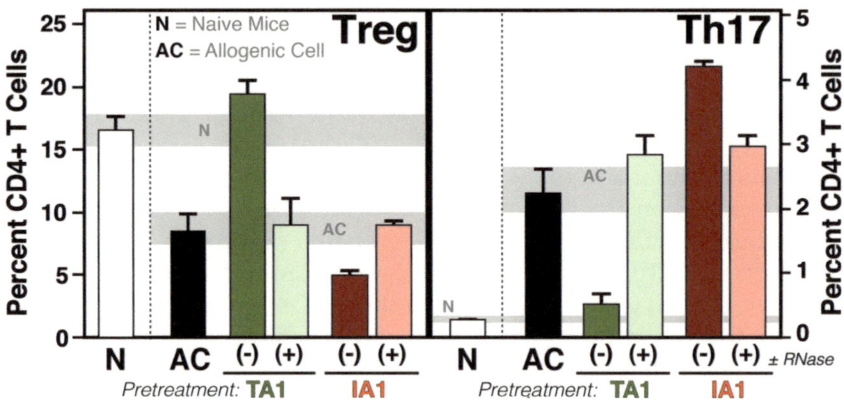

Figure 6.
The active component of TA1 and IA1 are miRNA as evidenced loss of immunomodulatory activity consequent to RNase treatment. A microRNA (miRNA) specific preparation made from mice previously treated (5 days prior) with mPEG-allogeneic leukocytes yielded a systemic immunomodulation (increased Tregs, decreased Th17 T cells) very similar to the mPEG-cellular product within the spleen of mice 5 days post treatment with the miRNA preparation. As shown, the immunomodulatory effect is lost by treatment with RNase enzymes. N = naïve mice; AC = allogeneic cells; miRNA alloplasma fraction ± RNase; and mPEG-alloplasma ± RNase.

6. Treatment of autoimmune diseases via Treg:Teff modulation

Autoimmunity arises consequent to an animal/individual's immune system recognizing their own tissues as *'non-self'*. The Non-Obese Diabetic (NOD) mouse is an inbred strain that exhibits the spontaneous development of a variety of autoimmune diseases including insulin dependent T1D. The murine autoimmune diabetes develops spontaneously around 16–20 weeks of age though studies indicate that the autoimmune process begins by weeks 3–4 [43–51]. Of note, the NOD mouse has been extensively used to study the mechanisms underlying autoimmune-mediated diabetes as well as to evaluate therapeutic interventions on disease pathogenesis. To investigate the ability of TA1 to attenuate disease progression and incidence, 7-week-old NOD mice were treated with TA1—no other interventions were done.

As demonstrated in **Figure 7A**, the onset and incidence of diabetes was assessed and correlated with the Treg:Teff ratio of the mice [31–35]. As shown, 75% of the untreated NOD mice, but only 40% of the TA1 treated mice, developed T1D. The onset of T1D was correlated with the Treg:Teff ratios of the individual mouse (Panel A). As shown, the TA1 treated mice exhibited significantly increased Treg: Teff ratio which correlated with significantly delayed onset of the disease in the mice that became diabetic. Mice with very high Treg:Teff ratios (average > 250) in either the control or TA1 treated mice remained normoglycemic. Moreover, TA-treatment was associated with improved islet histology (**Figure 7B**) as reflected by the lower incidence of overt insulitis and peri-insulitis. Indeed, no normal islets were observed in the control diabetic NOD mice. In contrast, in TA1 treated mice that became diabetic, almost 20% of their islets exhibited normal morphology—more than that observed in normoglycemic NOD mice at 30 weeks. In the normoglycemic TA1 treated mice > 40% of the islets exhibited normal histology.

Mechanistically, the changes noted in the Treg:Teff ratio (using $Foxp3^+$ and $Th17^+$ lymphocytes as surrogates for Treg and Teff, respectively) correlating with the changes noted in multiple T cell subsets [31]. As shown in **Figure 8**, analysis of the pancreatic lymph node demonstrated that TA1 induced multiple tolerogenic T cell subpopulations (e.g., $Foxp3^+$, $IL\text{-}10^+$, $TGF\text{-}\beta^+$ and $IL\text{-}4^+$ $CD4^+$ T cells) and down regulated multiple Teff subgroups ($Th17^+$, $IL\text{-}2^+$, $INF\text{-}\gamma^+$ and $TNF\text{-}\beta^+$ $CD4^+$ cells).

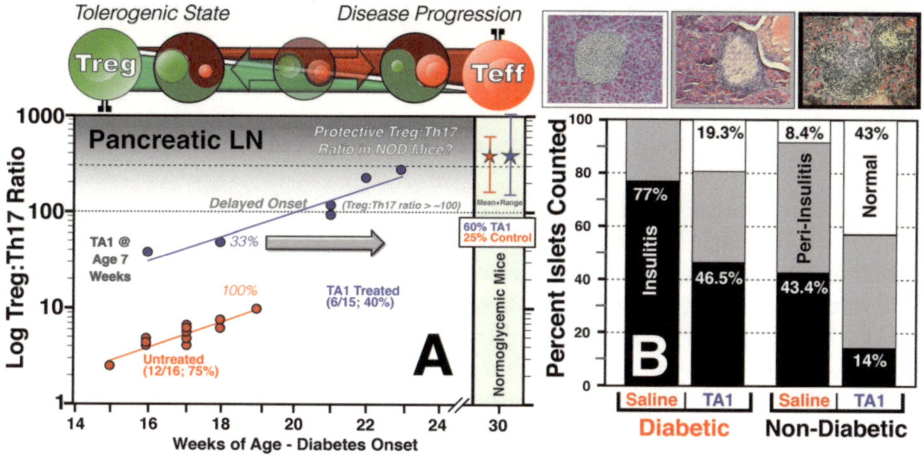

Figure 7.
Inhibition of T1D in the NOD mouse via induction of immunosuppression by the administration of immunomodulatory miRNA. Panel A: Age of onset for T1D versus the Treg:Teff ratio in the control and TA1-treated NOD mouse. Note that TA1 therapy dramatically increased the Treg:Teff ratio and delayed both onset and incidence of T1D. In contrast, in control NOD mice the Treg:Teff ratio shifted left towards the expansion of Teff cells and disease progression. Panel B: Shown are the percentages of pancreatic islets exhibiting normal morphology or evidence of insulitis or peri-insulitis. Also shown are photomicrographs of islets exhibiting (left to right) normal morphology, peri-insulitis and insulitis. Data from Wang et al. [31].

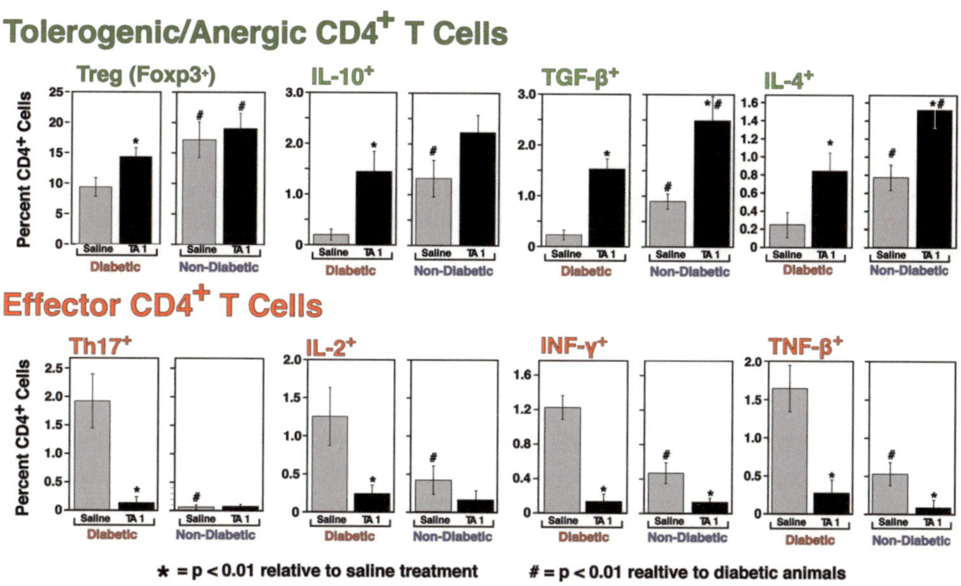

Figure 8.
Effect of TA1 therapy on T CD4+ T cell populations. As shown, TA1 therapy significantly increased multiple Treg populations in comparison to the control NOD mice. Concurrent with the increase in Treg subsets, TA1 very dramatically reduced the Teff subpopulations. The net consequence of TA1 therapy was a significant shift in the Treg:Teff ratio towards a tolerogenic state. Data from Wang et al. [31].

Hence, TA1 effectively skewed the Treg:Teff ratio towards a tolerogenic-immunosuppressive environment within the pancreas that consequently inhibited the effector T cell dependent autoimmune disease process. Importantly, the TA1 induced immunomodulation was not limited to the pancreas as T cell subtyping of multiple lymphoid tissues, as well and the blood, demonstrated that the induced tolerogenic environment was systemic in nature [31]. These systemic findings suggest that TA1 could be used to treat a broad range of T cell mediated autoimmune diseases.

7. Enhancing the anti-cancer response via Treg:Teff modulation

In contrast to autoimmune diseases, systemic immunosuppressive states can be highly problematic in the context of infectious agents (e.g., bacteria and viruses) and cancer. Indeed, this lack of immune response to cancer was the problem that Coley attempted to address with his immunomodulatory preparations. By injecting a toxic mixture, a broad immune response would be induced that, it was HOPED, would exert a non-specific bystander effect on cancer cells. This was, in fact, a relatively viable clinical approach as cancer cells tend to be more sensitive to metabolic (e.g., high fever, energy starvation) and immunological (e.g., T cell and complement activation) extremes. Indeed, *Coley's Toxins* were a mainstay of advanced cancer therapy for much of the early/mid twentieth century until their use was supplanted by *'safer'* radiation and chemo- therapy approaches. But *'safe'* is not always *'safe'*. The long-term toxicity effects of both radiation and chemotherapy are now becoming appreciated—especially when used in young patients. Hence, significant clinical efforts are now being directed towards increasingly expensive and labor/time intensive, immunotherapies that can either enhance the endogenous immune response to cancers or be engineered to attack specific cancers.

In contrast to these expensive and time-extensive cellular therapies, the bioproduction of IA1 (as well as TA1) is rapid and inexpensive. Moreover, minimal time (24 hours) is required to skew the Treg:Teff ratio of resting PBMC towards an inflammatory response arising from the simultaneous decrease of Treg and increase in Teff [34]. Hence IA1 could be used to enhance the immune response of autologous leukocytes thus obviating the risks associated with the adoptive transfer of allogenic T cells. Moreover, the strength of the inflammatory response is substantially less than that observed with other activation strategies (e.g., mitogens, anti-CD3, of allogeneic stimulation) reducing the risk of cytokine release syndrome [34]. Also, of potential value, the strength of the IA1 stimulation can, if necessary, be titrated using TA1.

To evaluate the potential anti-cancer efficacy of IA1 activated leukocytes, in vitro studies were conducted using HeLa and SH-4 melanoma cell lines (**Figure 9**) [34]. The direct toxicity and anti-proliferative effects of control and the SYN (prepared from resting cells) or IA1 treated PBMC against the HeLa (epithelial) and SH-4 (melanoma) human cancer cell lines were assessed using an ACEA iCELLigence (ACEA Biosciences, Inc., San Diego, CA). The iCELLigence provides a continuous, real-time, measurement of cell proliferation using changes in the electrical impedance within tissue culture wells. The change in impedance is induced by the increase in adherent cells and is unaffected by cells (e.g., PBMC) that remain non-adherent. All studies were done with an initial seeding density of 5000 HeLa, or 20,000 SH-4, cells per well. To assess the ability of SYN- or IA1-activation to enhance the anti-cancer efficacy of naïve lymphocytes, donor PBMC were pretreated with SYN or IA1 for 24 hours and then overlaid on seeded cancer cells at a ratio of 50 PBMC per cancer cell.

As shown, direct addition of IA1 to HeLa cells demonstrated that the IA1 therapeutic itself exhibited no direct effects on cancer cell proliferation (**Figure 9A**). However, when HeLa cells were overlaid with unactivated or SYN-activated allogenic donor PBMC, the T cells eventually recognized the allogenic HeLa cells and, after ~90 hours, inhibited cell proliferation and, ultimately, killed the HeLa cells as

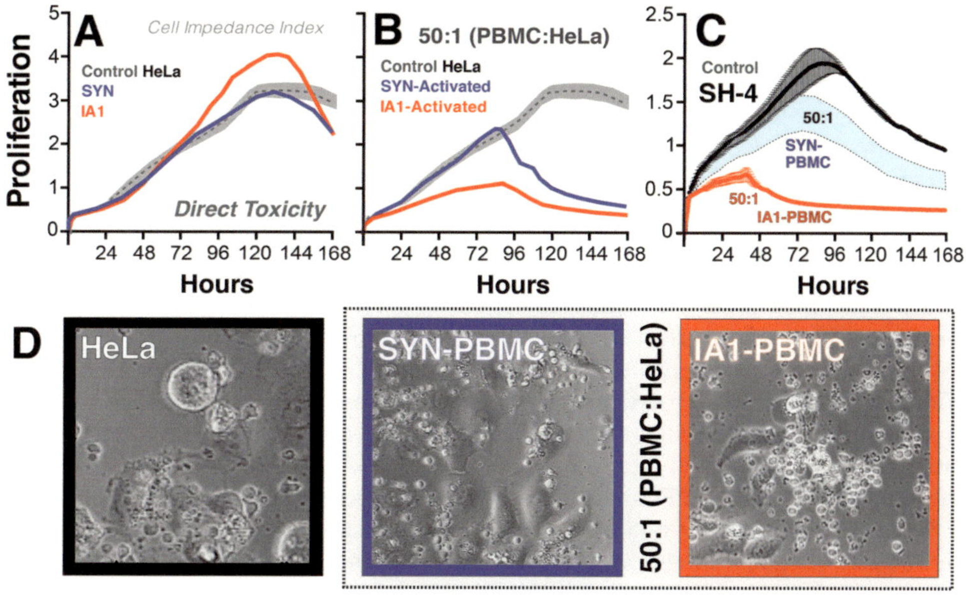

Figure 9.
IA1 enhances the anti-cancer efficacy of resting PBMC. Panel A: IA1 exhibits no direct toxicity to HeLa cells (shown) or PBMC (not shown). Panel B: IA-1 pre-treatment, but not SYN-pre-treatment, exhibited a greatly enhanced anti-cancer effect on HeLa cells. Panel C: Similarly to HeLa cells, IA1, but not SYN, pre-treated PBMC exhibited significant anti-SH-4 (melanoma) activity. Panel D: The enhanced efficacy of treated PBMC is supported by photomicrographs of allogenic PBMC responding to HeLa cells. As shown, after 72 hours incubation, resting unactivated PBMC show limited interaction when overlaid on HeLa cells. In contrast, the same PBMC, when treated for 24 hours with IA1, show a robust enhanced interaction with the HeLa cell monolayer. Cell proliferation was measured by changes in electrical impedance. SYN (derived from the secretome of resting PBMC) or IA1-pretreated utilized PBMC from the same donor. Modified from Yang et al. [34] and Scott et al. [35].

reflected by the decrease in the impedance index. In contrast, when IA1-activated PBMC were overlaid, the inhibition of HeLa cell proliferation was noted within the first 8–12 hours (versus ~90 hours) dramatically reducing the overall proliferation of the HeLa cells (**Figure 9B**). The anti-cancer efficacy of IA-activated PBMC was not limited to HeLa cells. Further studies using SH-4 melanoma cells also demonstrated that IA1-activation of naïve PBMC induced a potent anti-cancer effect (**Figure 9C**). As noted, control SH-4 melanoma cells showed rapid proliferation over 96 hours. However, when untreated SYN-pretreated PBMC (50 PBMC per SH-4 cell) were overlaid onto the seeded SH-4 cells at 0 hours, a significant, but modest, inhibition of SH-4 growth occurred. However, when IA1-pretreated (24 hours) PBMC from the same donor are overlaid on the SH-4 cells, a greatly enhanced anti-cancer effect was noted relative to untreated PBMC. The enhanced efficacy of treated PBMC was supported by photomicrographs of allogenic PBMC responding to HeLa cells (**Figure 9D**). As shown, after 72 hours incubation, SYN-activated PBMC exhibited limited interaction with the HeLa cells. In contrast, the same PBMC, when pre-treated for 24 hours with IA1, demonstrated a significantly enhanced interaction with the HeLa cell monolayer. Hence, in vitro, IA1 is capable of significantly enhancing the anti-cancer efficacy of resting PBMC. As such the secretome generated IA1 proved to be a potent adjuvant therapy for the activation of autologous lymphocytes in cancer patients. This approach could be done either by collection of PBMC with ex vivo activation for 24 hours, or as shown in **Figures 6–8**, direct systemic administration of the IA1-therapeutic to the patient. Moreover, this methodology could be used in conjunction with other ACT approaches.

8. Regulating the Treg:Teff ratio: toxicity and ping-pong immunology

Importantly, treatment of mice or cells with mPEG-splenocytes or the TA1 and IA1 (see **Figure 9A**) secretome products exerted no evidence of direct acute toxicity [27, 31, 34, 35]. Indeed, the safety of allogenic mPEG-splenocytes was demonstrated in a murine model of transfusion associated graft versus host disease in which it was shown that transfusion of mPEG-splenocytes were incapable of inducing graft versus host disease in immunocompromise (irradiated) mice [25]. This is not to say that these approaches may not be prone to chronic side effects. Immunosuppressive therapy, i.e., tolerization, is known to increase the risk of cancer. Thus, the long-term persistence of the effects of mPEG-leukocytes or TA1 [35] could pose a similar risk. Indeed, our previous studies have demonstrated that the immunomodulatory effects of both the PEGylated allogenic splenocytes and the TA1 and IA1 secretome products extend well beyond the circulation time of donor lymphocytes and exhibit functional activity both in vitro and in vivo [27, 31, 33–35]. For example, in mice treated with allogenic mPEG-splenocytes, the Tregs remained significantly elevated at 30 days post treatment and, when challenged with a secondary transfusion of unmodified allogenic splenocytes, prevented the expected (decreased Treg and increased Teff) proinflammatory effects of the allogenic splenocyte transfusion.

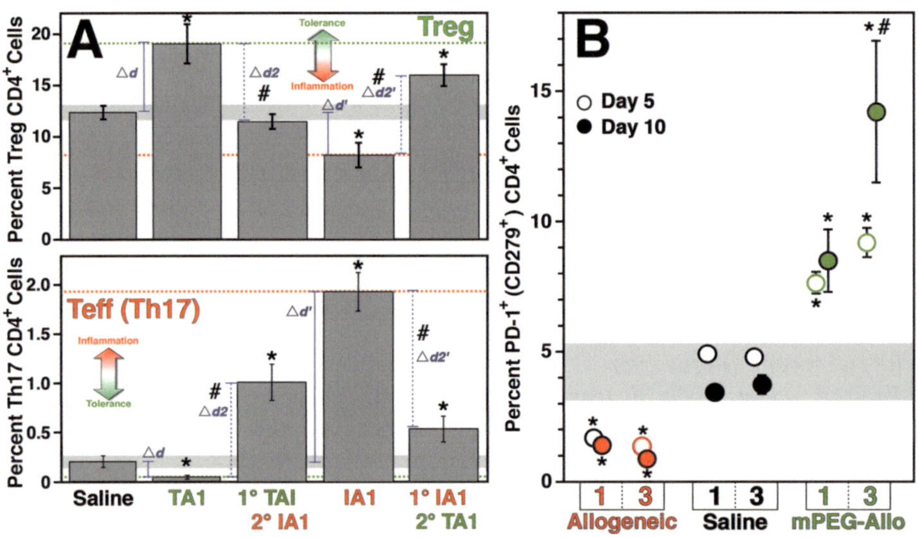

Figure 10.
*Ping-pong immunology of TA1 and IA1. Panel A: Shown are the Treg (Foxp3⁺) and Teff (Th17) CD4⁺ cells in the spleen of mice treated with a primary (1°) infusion of either TA1 or IA1. A subset of mice were subsequently received a secondary (2°) infusion with the opposing therapeutic (IA1 or TA1) at day 9. Lymphoid organs (spleen shown) were harvested at day 40. As noted by the absolute percentage of CD4⁺ T cells and the delta ( ) d/d' from naïve mice, primary (1°) treatment with TA1 and IA1 alone gave the expected Treg and Teff response. The 2° treatment with the opposite miRNA preparation was able to significantly counterbalance the effect of the 1° treatment. This is reflected by the d2 and d2' bars and the regression of the Treg and Th17 values towards the mean of naïve mice. As expected based on the magnitude of the 1° treatment, the d2 and d2' bars were greater than the initial d/d' values. This is most obvious with the Th17 cells where both the magnitude and actual decrease in the 2° d2 (~1.5%) for TA1 was significantly greater than 1° d (~0.15%). Panel B: PD-1⁺ (CD279⁺) CD4⁺ T cells are important in downregulating the immune response and promoting self-tolerance via suppression of Teff cell populations. As shown, transfusion of allogeneic splenocytes downregulated, while mPEG-allogenic splenocytes upregulated, PD-1⁺ cells relative to naïve, saline treated, mice. Shown are the PD-1⁺ cells in the spleen of mice treated with a primary (1°) infusion of either allogenic or mPEG-allogenic at day 0 (denoted as 1) or a total of 3 injections given at days 0, 2 and 4 (denoted as 3). Spleens were harvested at either day 5 or 10 for determination of T cell subpopulations. N ≥ 5 for all samples shown. Significance: * $p < 0.01$ from naïve mice; # $p < 0.01$ from primary TA1 or IA1 (panel a) or; panel B from 1 or 3 doses.*

Indeed, the Treg remained high and no Th17 cells were induced [27]. Long-term studies of mice treated once with TA1 also demonstrated a persistent, and significant, elevation in their Treg cells for ≥270 days [35]. Hence, the potent immunomodulatory effects of this approach could be of concern.

As noted above, the persistence of the Treg response, even upon allogenic challenge, while beneficial in the treatment of autoimmune diseases could pose immunological risks. However, TA1 and IA1 target the same miRNA-based bioregulatory pathway governing lymphocyte differentiation and proliferation. Because of this, TA1 and IA1 are capable of counter-acting the activity of the other. This *'ping-pong immunology'* in mice is demonstrated in **Figure 10A**. As noted, treatment with TA1 or IA1 inversely affects the Treg and Teff populations (Δd, Δd'). However, subsequent administration of the IA1 to TA1 treated mice, or vise-versa, resulted in the Treg and Teff cell populations reverting towards the homeostatic level noted in naïve, untreated, mice (Δd2, Δd2'). The immunomodulatory *'ping-pong'* activity of TA1 and IA1 can be further fine-tuned via dosing, as both TA1 and IA1 show dose dependent activity [31–35]. Also of note, the immunomodulatory activity of this technology is correlated with other markers of tolerance or inflammation. Transfusion of mPEG-splenocytes triggers a significant upregulation of $PD\text{-}1^{+}$ (CD279) $CD4^{+}$ lymphocytes (**Figure 10B**). These $PD\text{-}1^{+}$ cells are important in downregulating the immune response and promoting self-tolerance via suppression of Teff cell populations. The expression of $PD\text{-}1^{+}$ T cells may underlie the production of $IL\text{-}10^{+}$ T cells as noted in **Figure 8**. In contrast to TA1 treatment, both unmodified allogenic cells (shown) and IA1 treatment (not shown) decrease PD-1 expression relative to naïve mice. A dose effect on PD-1 expression can be seen with both allogenic and, especially, mPEG-allogenic cells in mice receiving 1 or 3 injections (at days 0, 2 and 4) of cells when assessed at days 5 and 10 post treatment.

9. Conclusions

Immunosuppression and immunoactivation represent the divergent ends of the Treg:Teff ratio continuum (**Figure 1**). While pharmacologic agents have historically been the primary tools for modulating the Teff response, few options have existed for modulating (especially upregulating) the Treg response. However, the direct immunomodulation of the endogenous immune system may have significant clinical benefit in treating a broad range of clinical conditions ranging from autoimmune diseases, tissue/organ engraftment, and cancer. Extensive in vitro and in vivo studies in our laboratory have demonstrated that PEGylated lymphocytes as well as the biomanufactured TA1 and IA1 exhibited significant immunomodulatory activity [23–42, 52]. Indeed, these agents directly altered the Treg:Teff ratio by simultaneously modulating both regulatory and effector T cell subsets. Consequent to their immunomodulatory activity, the immunosuppressive TA1 therapeutic significantly delayed the onset and overall incidence of autoimmune diabetes in the NOD mouse [31]. Conversely, the proinflammatory IA1 therapeutic directly activated T cells overcoming their inherent immunological inertia resulting in enhanced recognition and killing of cancer cells [34]. The immunomodulatory effects of these agents were highly persistent [35]. The TA1 and IA1 agents showed dose dependency and could be used to counteract the effect of on another [31–35]. The successful development of these immunomodulatory therapeutics may prove useful in facilitating organ engraftment, treating autoimmune disease and enhancing the endogenous anti-cancer response.

Acknowledgements

The authors would like to thank Wendy Toyofuku and Drs. Duncheng Wang and Ning Kang for their past contributions to the work presented in this chapter. This work was supported by grants from the Canadian Institutes of Health Research (Grant No. 123317; MDS), Canadian Blood Services (MDS) and Health Canada (MDS). The views expressed herein do not necessarily represent the view of the federal government of Canada. We thank the Canada Foundation for Innovation and the Michael Smith Foundation for Health Research for infrastructure funding at the University of British Columbia Centre for Blood Research. The funders had no role in study design, data collection and analysis, decision to publish, or preparation of the manuscript.

Conflict of interest

Canadian Blood Services is pursuing patents related to the production and utilization of the described acellular immunomodulatory agents. Canadian Blood Services, a not-for-profit organization responsible for collecting, manufacturing and distributing blood and blood products to all Canadians (except Quebec), is the assignee for relevant patents. MDS is an inventor on these patents. XY has no conflicts of interests.

Author details

Xining Yang[1] and Mark D. Scott[2,3,4*]

1 Terry Fox Laboratory, British Columbia Cancer, Vancouver, Canada

2 Centre for Innovation, Canadian Blood Services, University of British Columbia, Vancouver, Canada

3 Centre for Blood Research, University of British Columbia, Vancouver, Canada

4 Department of Pathology and Laboratory Medicine, University of British Columbia, Vancouver, Canada

*Address all correspondence to: mdscott@mail.ubc.ca

References

[1] Steinmetz M, Hood L. Genes of the major histocompatibility complex in mouse and man. Science. 1983;**222**: 727-733. DOI: 10.1126/science.6356354

[2] Trivedi VB, Dave AP, Dave JM, Patel BC. Human leukocyte antigen and its role in transplantation biology. Transplantation Proceedings. 2007;**39**: 688-693. DOI: 10.1016/j.transproceed. 2007.01.066

[3] Spierings E, Fleischhauer K. Histocompatibility. In: Carreras E, Dufour C, Mohty M, Kröger N, editors. The EBMT Handbook: Hematopoietic Stem Cell Transplantation and Cellular Therapies. Cham (CH): Springer; 2019

[4] Suntharalingam G, Perry MR, Ward S, et al. Cytokine storm in a phase 1 trial of the anti-CD28 monoclonal antibody TGN1412. The New England Journal of Medicine. 2006;**355**: 1018-1028. DOI: 10.1056/NEJMoa063842

[5] Hod EA, Cadwell CM, Liepkalns JS, et al. Cytokine storm in a mouse model of IgG-mediated hemolytic transfusion reactions. Blood. 2008;**112**:891-894. DOI: 10.1182/blood-2008-01-132092

[6] Bonifant CL, Jackson HJ, Brentjens RJ, Curran KJ. Toxicity and management in CAR T-cell therapy. Molecular Therapy Oncolytics. 2016;**3**: 16011. DOI: 10.1038/mto.2016.11

[7] Chen H, Wang F, Zhang P, Zhang Y, Chen Y, Fan X, et al. Management of cytokine release syndrome related to CAR-T cell therapy. Frontiers in Medicine. 2019;**13**:610-617. DOI: 10.1007/s11684-019-0714-8

[8] Coley WB. The treatment of inoperable sarcoma by bacterial toxins (the mixed toxins of the *Streptococcus erysipelas* and the *Bacillus prodigiosus*). Proceedings of the Royal Society of Medicine. 1910;**3**:1-48

[9] Coley WB. IX. Contribution to the study of sarcoma of the femur: Periosteal round-celled sarcoma of the femur, involving two-thirds of the shaft, with very extensive multiple metastases-apparent cure by the mixed toxins of erysipelas and *Bacillus prodigiosus*. Well 10(1/2) years, when a malignant tumor (sarcoma and epithelioma) developed in the thigh at the site of an old X-ray dermatitis. Annals of Surgery. 1913;**58**:97-108. DOI: 10.1097/00000658-191307000-00010

[10] Coley WB. The treatment of malignant tumors by repeated inoculations of erysipelas. With a report of ten original cases 1893. Clinical Orthopaedics and Related Research. 1991:3-11

[11] Starnes CO. Coley's toxins in perspective. Nature. 1992;**357**:11-12. DOI: 10.1038/357011a0

[12] Frahm M, Felgner S, Kocijancic D, et al. Efficiency of conditionally attenuated *Salmonella enterica* serovar Typhimurium in bacterium-mediated tumor therapy. MBio. 2015;**6**:1-11. DOI: 10.1128/mBio.00254-15

[13] Zheng JH, Nguyen VH, Jiang SN, et al. Two-step enhanced cancer immunotherapy with engineered *Salmonella typhimurium* secreting heterologous flagellin. Science Translational Medicine. 2017;**9**:eaak9537. DOI: 10.1126/scitranslmed.aak9537

[14] Desjardins A, Gromeier M, Herndon JE, et al. Recurrent glioblastoma treated with recombinant poliovirus. The New England Journal of Medicine. 2018;**379**:150-161. DOI: 10.1056/NEJMoa1716435

[15] Schulof RS, Mai D, Nelson MA, et al. Active specific immunotherapy with an autologous tumor cell vaccine in

patients with resected non-small cell lung cancer. Molecular Biotherapy. 1988;**1**:30-36

[16] Ockert D, Schirrmacher V, Beck N, et al. Newcastle disease virus-infected intact autologous tumor cell vaccine for adjuvant active specific immunotherapy of resected colorectal carcinoma. Clinical Cancer Research. 1996;**2**:21-28

[17] Baars A, van Riel JM, Cuesta MA, Jaspars EH, Pinedo HM, van den Eertwegh AJ. Metastasectomy and active specific immunotherapy for a large single melanoma metastasis. Hepato-Gastroenterology. 2002;**49**: 691-693

[18] Berger M, Kreutz FT, Horst JL, Baldi AC, Koff WJ. Phase I study with an autologous tumor cell vaccine for locally advanced or metastatic prostate cancer. Journal of Pharmacy & Pharmaceutical Sciences. 2007;**10**: 144-152

[19] Fishman M, Hunter TB, Soliman H, et al. Phase II trial of B7-1 (CD-86) transduced, cultured autologous tumor cell vaccine plus subcutaneous interleukin-2 for treatment of stage IV renal cell carcinoma. Journal of Immunotherapy. 2008;**31**:72-80. DOI: 10.1097/CJI.0b013e31815ba792

[20] D'Aloia MM, Zizzari IG, Sacchetti B, Pierelli L, Alimandi M. CAR-T cells: The long and winding road to solid tumors. Cell Death & Disease. 2018;**9**:282. DOI: 10.1038/s41419-018-0278-6

[21] Mullard A. FDA approves first CAR T therapy. Nature Reviews. Drug Discovery. 2017;**16**:669. DOI: 10.1038/nrd.2017.196

[22] Bach PB, Giralt SA, Saltz LB. FDA approval of Tisagenlecleucel: Promise and complexities of a $475 000 cancer drug. Journal of the American Medical Association. 2017;**318**:1861-1862. DOI: 10.1001/jama.2017.15218

[23] Murad KL, Gosselin EJ, Eaton JW, Scott MD. Stealth cells: Prevention of major histocompatibility complex class II-mediated T-cell activation by cell surface modification. Blood. 1999;**94**: 2135-2141

[24] Chen AM, Scott MD. Current and future applications of immunological attenuation via pegylation of cells and tissue. BioDrugs. 2001;**15**:833-847. DOI: 10.2165/00063030-200115120-00005

[25] Chen AM, Scott MD. Immunocamouflage: Prevention of transfusion-induced graft-versus-host disease via polymer grafting of donor cells. Journal of Biomedical Materials Research. Part A. 2003;**67**:626-636

[26] Chen AM, Scott MD. Comparative analysis of polymer and linker chemistries on the efficacy of immunocamouflage of murine leukocytes. Artificial Cells, Blood Substitutes, and Immobilization Biotechnology. 2006;**34**:305-322. DOI: 10.1080/10731190600683845

[27] Wang D, Toyofuku WM, Chen AM, Scott MD. Induction of immunotolerance via mPEG grafting to allogeneic leukocytes. Biomaterials. 2011;**32**: 9494-9503. DOI: 10.1016/j.biomaterials. 2011.08.061

[28] Wang D, Toyofuku WM, Scott MD. The potential utility of methoxypoly (ethylene glycol)-mediated prevention of rhesus blood group antigen RhD recognition in transfusion medicine. Biomaterials. 2012;**33**:3002-3012. DOI: 10.1016/j.biomaterials.2011.12.041

[29] Wang D, Toyofuku WM, Kyluik DL, Scott MD. Use of flow cytometry in the in vitro and in vivo analysis of tolerance/anergy induction by immunocamouflage. In: Schmid I, editor. Flow Cytometry-Recent

Perspectives. Croatia: IntechOpen; 2012. pp. 133-150

[30] Kyluik-Price DL, Li L, Scott MD. Comparative efficacy of blood cell immunocamouflage by membrane grafting of methoxypoly(ethylene glycol) and polyethyloxazoline. Biomaterials. 2014;**35**:412-422. DOI: 10.1016/j.biomaterials.2013.09.016

[31] Wang D, Shanina I, Toyofuku WM, Horwitz MS, Scott MD. Inhibition of autoimmune diabetes in NOD mice by miRNA therapy. PLoS One. 2015;**10**: e0145179. DOI: 10.1371/journal.pone.0145179

[32] Kyluik-Price DL, Scott MD. Effects of methoxypoly (ethylene glycol) mediated immunocamouflage on leukocyte surface marker detection, cell conjugation, activation and alloproliferation. Biomaterials. 2016;**74**: 167-177. DOI: 10.1016/j.biomaterials.2015.09.047

[33] Kang N, Toyofuku WM, Yang X, Scott MD. Inhibition of allogeneic cytotoxic T cell (CD8(+)) proliferation via polymer-induced Treg (CD4(+)) cells. Acta Biomaterialia. 2017;**57**: 146-155. DOI: 10.1016/j.actbio.2017.04.025

[34] Yang X, Kang N, Toyofuku WM, Scott MD. Enhancing the pro-inflammatory anti-cancer T cell response via biomanufactured, secretome-based, immunotherapeutics. Immunobiology. 2018;**224**:270-284. DOI: 10.1016/j.imbio.2018.12.003

[35] Scott MD, Wang D, Toyofuku WM, Yang X. Modulating the T lymphocyte immune response via Secretome produced miRNA: From tolerance induction to the enhancement of the anticancer response. In: Cells of the Immune System. Croatia: IntechOpen; 2019

[36] Scott MD, Murad KL. Cellular camouflage: Fooling the immune system with polymers. Current Pharmaceutical Design. 1998;**4**:423-438

[37] Scott MD, Bradley AJ, Murad KL. Camouflaged blood cells: Low-technology bioengineering for transfusion medicine? Transfusion Medicine Reviews. 2000;**14**:53-63. DOI: 10.1016/S0887-7963(00)80115-7

[38] Scott MD, Chen AM. Beyond the red cell: Pegylation of other blood cells and tissues. Transfusion Clinique et Biologique. 2004;**11**:40-46. DOI: 10.1016/j.tracli.2003.12.005

[39] Bradley AJ, Scott MD. Immune complex binding by immunocamouflaged [poly(ethylene glycol)-grafted] erythrocytes. American Journal of Hematology. 2007;**82**: 970-975. DOI: 10.1002/ajh.20956

[40] Le Y, Scott MD. Immunocamouflage: The biophysical basis of immunoprotection by grafted methoxypoly(ethylene glycol) (mPEG). Acta Biomaterialia. 2010;**6**:2631-2641. DOI: 10.1016/j.actbio.2010.01.031

[41] Wang D, Kyluik DL, Murad KL, Toyofuku WM, Scott MD. Polymer-mediated immunocamouflage of red blood cells: Effects of polymer size on antigenic and immunogenic recognition of allogeneic donor blood cells. Science China. Life Sciences. 2011;**54**:589-598. DOI: 10.1007/s11427-011-4190-x

[42] Le Y, Li L, Wang D, Scott MD. Immunocamouflage of latex surfaces by grafted methoxypoly(ethylene glycol) (mPEG): Proteomic analysis of plasma protein adsorption. Science China. Life Sciences. 2012;**55**:191-201. DOI: 10.1007/s11427-012-4290-2

[43] Anderson MS, Bluestone JA. The NOD mouse: A model of immune dysregulation. Annual Review of Immunology. 2005;**23**:447-485. DOI: 10.1146/annurev.immunol.23.021704.115643

[44] Haskins K. Pathogenic T-cell clones in autoimmune diabetes: More lessons from the NOD mouse. Advances in Immunology. 2005;**87**:123-162. DOI: 10.1016/S0065-2776(05)87004-X

[45] Thayer TC, Wilson SB, Mathews CE. Use of nonobese diabetic mice to understand human type 1 diabetes. Endocrinology and Metabolism Clinics of North America. 2010;**39**:541-561. DOI: 10.1016/j.ecl.2010.05.001

[46] Horwitz MS, Ilic A, Fine C, Rodriguez E, Sarvetnick N. Coxsackievirus-mediated hyperglycemia is enhanced by reinfection and this occurs independent of T cells. Virology. 2003;**314**:510-520. DOI: 10.1016/S0042-6822(03)00462-8

[47] Horwitz MS, Knudsen M, Ilic A, Fine C, Sarvetnick N. Transforming growth factor-beta inhibits coxsackievirus-mediated autoimmune myocarditis. Viral Immunology. 2006; **19**:722-733. DOI: 10.1089/vim.2006.19.722

[48] Richer MJ, Horwitz MS. Viral infections in the pathogenesis of autoimmune diseases: Focus on type 1 diabetes. Frontiers in Bioscience. 2008; **13**:4241-4257

[49] Richer MJ, Horwitz MS. Coxsackievirus infection as an environmental factor in the etiology of type 1 diabetes. Autoimmunity Reviews. 2009;**8**:611-615. DOI: 10.1016/j.autrev.2009.02.006

[50] Richer MJ, Horwitz MS. Preventing viral-induced type 1 diabetes. Annals of the New York Academy of Sciences. 2009;**1173**:487-492. DOI: 10.1111/j.1749-6632.2009.04662.x

[51] Richer MJ, Straka N, Fang D, Shanina I, Horwitz MS. Regulatory T-cells protect from type 1 diabetes after induction by coxsackievirus infection in the context of transforming growth factor-beta. Diabetes. 2008;**57**: 1302-1311. DOI: 10.2337/db07-1460

[52] Scott MD, Bradley AJ, Murad KL. Stealth erythrocytes: Effects of polymer grafting on biophysical, biological and immunological parameters. Blood Transfusion. 2003;**1**:244-265

Chapter 3

Novel Diagnostic and Therapeutic Approach to Antibody-Mediated Rejections in Heart Transplantation

Takuya Watanabe and Norihide Fukushima

Abstract

Despite the improvement of immunosuppressive therapy in heart transplantation (HTx), antibody-mediated rejection (AMR) is still a great obstacle to prolong cardiac graft survival. Anti-donor-specific antibodies (DSAs), especially anti-donor human leukocyte antigen (HLA) antibody, lead to heart graft failure resulting in hemodynamic consequence and often in the recipient death. To prevent hyperacute rejection, prospective complement-dependent cytotoxicity test has been performed in every cardiac donor in Japan. But in other solid organ transplantations, flow cytometry crossmatch has been recently recommended to crossmatch to select the recipient in Japan as well as the world. However, flow cytometry is too sensitive to select the recipient, because not all DSAs determined by flow cytometry are cytotoxic to the cardiac graft. On the first complement classical pathway, alloantibodies bind to HLA antigens on cells of the graft and then recruit C1q, which is essential to make membrane attack complex and kill the cell. We review a role of the novel monitoring method of complement pathway regarding C1q in occurrence of AMR and its diagnostic and therapeutic significance in managing AMR in HTx.

Keywords: heart transplantation, antibody-mediated rejection, sensitization, complement binding donor-specific antibodies, C1q assay

1. Introduction

Although immunosuppressive therapy in heart transplantation (HTx) has been remarkably improved, antibody-mediated rejection (AMR) is still a great obstacle to prolong cardiac graft survival [1, 2]. AMR may develop when recipient antibodies against donor human leukocyte antigen (HLA) on the endothelial cells exist in the recipient serum [3]. The presence of circulating anti-donor-specific antibodies (DSAs) has several impacts on clinical outcomes both before and after HTx. The timing of sensitization against DSAs can be divided into the pre- and posttransplant periods [4]. The standard method to detect preformed antibodies at the time of HTx has been the complement-dependent cytotoxicity (CDC) test using recipient serum and donor leukocytes [5]. In Japan, only the donor heart with negative prospective CDC crossmatching with T lymphocytes has been transplanted, and none of 512 HTx consecutive recipients transplanted between 1999 and 2019 in Japan experienced hyperacute rejection (HAR) [6]. Although flow cytometry has been recently recommended to crossmatch to select the recipient in the world in solid organ transplantation, flow cytometry is too sensitive to select the recipient, because not all DSAs determined by flow cytometry are always cytotoxic to the cardiac graft cells [7–9]. Posttransplant antibodies produced before and after HTx are currently screened for evaluating AMR development using single antigen Luminex bead (SAB) assay or panel reactive antibodies (PRA) test to detect DSAs in the recipient serum. However, their clinical impact is not clear and may be less elucidated in HTx. Further optimal protocol for management strategies for AMR to reflect clinical prognosis is needed [4, 9]. A detection of circulating complement binding DSAs may be promising. We review the role of the novel management method using complement binding ability assay in prevention, diagnosis, therapy, and monitoring of AMR in HTx.

2. Overview of AMR in HTx

HAR, the immediate form of AMR may occur within 0 to a few days after HTx if a certain level of preformed DSAs exists in the recipient serum. Early AMR may occur during the first month, usually within 1 or 2 weeks after HTx because of newly production of de novo DSAs or enhanced production of preformed DSAs. These early type AMRs are usually associated with allograft dysfunction and hemodynamic compromise [2–4, 9–11]. Late AMR may occur months to years after HTx, most likely due to enhanced recognition [10, 12–15]. Approximately 50% of HTx recipients who develop rejection later than 7 years after HTx are associated with evidence of AMR [16]. Up to 24% of cases with late AMR has been reported concurrent with cellular rejection [17]. As more sensitive diagnostic tools have become available for detecting AMR in HTx, the evidence that AMR is a wide spectrum of immunologic injury that ranges from subclinical, histological, immunologic, serological findings and/or graft dysfunction was increased [4, 9, 18].

2.1 Clinical features and diagnosis of AMR in HTx

2.1.1 Hyperacute rejection in HTx

HAR is a rare cause of primary cardiac graft failure occurring within minutes to hours of aortic unclamping with a high mortality rate of around 70% in HTx [19, 20]. Preformed antibodies directed against donor HLA class I antigens or ABO antigen expressed on the donor vascular endothelium mediate complement deposition with widespread hemorrhage and thrombosis within the cardiac allograft [20]. HLA class II molecules are not usually expressed on the donor vasculature, but they can be induced by inflammation and injury associated with procurement and preservation of the heart graft. At last, antibodies against non-HLA endothelial antigens may also lead to HAR. Previous blood product transfusions (particularly platelets), mechanical circulatory support (MCS), pregnancy, and previous transplantation may increase the likelihood of the presence of preformed DSAs. The use of leukocyte-depleted transfusions may decrease the risk for DSA production. To prevent HAR, CDC PRA screening is used to determine the presence of circulating DSAs [5]. In Japan, by routinely performing prospective CDC crossmatching with T lymphocytes since the first HTx in 1999, no HTx recipients experienced HAR [6]. A higher PRA is associated with worse AMR rates and poorer overall survival [21]. In patients with a high percentage of PRAs (>10%), perioperative plasmapheresis combined with immunoglobulin therapy may be used to reduce the incidence and severity of HAR. These interventions have allowed for transplantation between donors and recipients with positive crossmatches. HAR is manifested as severe biventricular failure that, if immediate re-HTx cannot be carried out, is usually fatal [4, 9, 20].

Grade	Definition	Substrates
pAMR 0	Negative for pathological AMR	Histological and immunopathologic studies are both negative
pAMR 1 (H+)	Histologic AMR alone	Histological findings present, and immunopathologic findings are negative
pAMR (I+)	Immunopathologic AMR alone	Histologic findings are negative, and immunopathologic findings are positive (CD68+ and/or C4d+)
pAMR2	Pathologic AMR	Histologic and immunopathologic findings are both present
pAMR3	Severe pathologic AMR	Interstitial hemorrhage, capillary fragmentation, mixed inflammatory infiltrates, endothelial cell pyknosis, and/or karyorrhexis and marked edema and immunopathologic findings are present. These cases may be associated with profound hemodynamic dysfunction and poor clinical outcomes

AMR, antibody-mediated rejection; pAMR, pathological AMR.

Table 1.
Recent novel diagnosis criteria in immunopathologic features.

2.1.2 Acute antibody-mediated rejection in HTx

Symptoms of acute AMR are those of right and left ventricular systolic and diastolic dysfunction and include exertion dyspnea, orthopnea, paroxysmal nocturnal dyspnea, high jugular venous pressure, edema, and abdominal distention. In infants, those can include feeding intolerance, irritability, and poor body weight gain. Acute AMR is associated with hemodynamic compromise in 10–47% of cases [2, 4, 9, 18]. The symptoms and signs of hemodynamic compromise have been highly variable, and the spectrum of cardiac graft dysfunction may range from decreased ejection fraction to cardiogenic shock requiring inotropic support and/or MCS [18].

2.2 Pathological diagnosis of AMR

Although multiple imaging tools have been developed in the detection of AMR as well as cellular rejection, the best diagnostic strategies for AMR have not been established. Therefore, endomyocardial biopsy (EMB) remains the "gold standard" for establishing the diagnosis of AMR. Recent novel diagnosis criteria for AMR consist of immunopathologic criteria (**Table 1**) in addition to the clinical manifestation of AMR [3, 19].

3. Management of AMR

3.1 Preventive method related to AMR

3.1.1 Desensitization strategies

Specific preventive strategies are needed to enable successful HTx in highly sensitized patients, because the presence of DSAs reduces the chance to obtain compatible donors, extends waiting times to HTx, increases the risk of mortality during awaiting HTx, and raises the risks of acute AMR and cardiac allograft vasculopathy after HTx [22]. Despite the emergent application of the promising agents such as bortezomib which is a 26S proteasome inhibitor and eculizumab which is a recombinant anti-C5 monoclonal antibody, a significant knowledge discrepancy remains with the current data for desensitization, investigated mostly from non-heart organ living donor transplants [23–28] and small observational studies in HTx [29–32]. The ideal desensitization strategy remains elusive especially in the HTx field. Moreover, clinical modalities to evaluate the efficacy of desensitization therapy are limited. Importantly, long-term outcomes and cost-effectiveness of desensitization strategies in HTx have not been well evaluated [4, 9].

3.1.2 Recipient selection in patients with preformed DSAs

As CDC assay is most clinically relevant methods for preventing accelerated early AMR as well as HAR in HTx [4, 9] but needs the technical expertise and experience, in many countries, before transplantation, the potential recipient is screened for circulating anti-HLA antibodies by using SAB assay or PRA test. If the percentage of PRA test is greater than 5–15%, most cardiac transplant centers require a negative prospective crossmatch between donor and recipient sera. However, the requirement for prospective crossmatch, which delays organ harvesting, may remarkably prolong a recipient's waiting time. On the other hand, in Japan, prospective CDC crossmatching with T lymphocytes has been routinely performed and completely avoided HAR since HTx program was started in 1999 [6]. But HTx must avoid false negatives because graft failure due to HAR may be directly life-threatening, so might need more sensitive tests.

3.2 Therapeutic method of AMR

3.2.1 Treatment of hyperacute rejection

According to the ISTH guideline 2016 [18], treatment for HAR should be initiated as soon as the diagnosis is defined, even when the patient is still in the operating room. Treatments for HAR include (1) high-dose intravenous (IV) corticosteroid (CS); (2) plasmapheresis; (3) IV immunoglobulin (IVIg); (4) cytolytic immunosuppressive therapy, such as antithymocyte or lymphocyte globulin; (5) calcineurin inhibitor (CNI) [cyclosporine (CYA) and tacrolimus (Tac)] and metabolic cycle inhibitors (i.e., mycophenolate mofetil; MMF); (6) IV inotropes and vasopressors; and (7) MCS.

Intraoperative myocardial biopsy is strongly recommended to confirm the diagnosis of HAR. Urgent re-HTx may be considered if the above therapies do not restore adequate cardiac graft function, but re-HTx for HAR has a considerably high mortality rate.

3.2.2 Treatment of acute antibody rejection (AMR)

Guidelines for treatment have recently been recommended by the ISHLT 2016 [18]. *Class II a* recommendations are followed.

1. To restore the immune-mediated cardiac graft injury in AMR: (1) high-dose IV CS and (2) cytolytic immunosuppressive therapy

2. To reduce circulating DSAs or their reactivity: (1) plasmapheresis, (2) immune apheresis (immunoadsorption), and (3) IVIg

3. To keep adequate hemodynamics: (1) IV inotropes and vasopressors and (2) MCS

4. When AMR is suspected, immunohistochemistry stains for complement split products (i.e., C4d) and possibly antibody should be added to standard histologic examination for EMB

5. The presence, quantity, and specificity of DSAs in the recipient serum should be screened

6. Follow-up EMB including immunohistochemistry staining should be performed 1–4 weeks after initiation of therapy

7. Maintenance immunosuppressive therapy after AMR treatment may be adjusted: (1) increase in the dose of current immunosuppressive agent(s), (2) addition of new agent(s), and (3) conversion to different agent(s) as shown below

Class II b recommendations are followed.

1. Systemic anticoagulation may reduce intravascular thrombosis in the cardiac allograft

2. Emergent re-HTx may be considered if the above therapies do not restore adequate cardiac graft function, but prognosis in this situation is poor

The benefit of treating subclinical AMR has not been elucidated. AMR might be a clinical-pathological continuation which starts with a latent immunological response of circulating DSAs with C4d deposition without clinical or histological changes, to a subclinical AMR, and finally to symptomatic AMR. A recent consensus recommends treating AMR in the presence of graft dysfunction regardless of histopathological finding, pAMR 2 in the absence of graft dysfunction if DSAs possibly relevant to AMR are present, and pAMR 3 regardless of the clinical findings [18].

3.2.3 Maintenance immunosuppressive strategies after treating AMR

The principles for the post-AMR management consist of reducing circulating DSAs and suppressing production of additional DSAs and T- and B-lymphocyte responses. However, currently there are only recommendations based on consensus [18].

The current available therapies are as follows: (1) suppression of the T-lymphocyte response (i.e., CS, MMF, cytolytic immunosuppressive therapy, photopheresis, or total lymphoid irradiation), (2) depletion of circulating DSAs (i.e., plasmapheresis), (3) suppression of residual DSAs (i.e., IVIg), (4) depletion of B lymphocytes (i.e., CS, rituximab, or splenectomy), (5) depletion of plasma cells (i.e., bortezomib), and (6) suppression of complement (i.e., eculizumab, IVIg).

4. What are the methods of detecting DSAs most relevant to clinical outcomes?

AMR in HTx is caused by the complex pathogenesis and immunopathologic pathway [2–4, 9, 18]. AMR develops when recipient serum contains DSAs against the endothelial layer of the cardiac allograft. Antibodies bind complement and activate the complement cascade, resulting in endothelial and myocardial injury. Complements, its fragments, and immunoglobulin are deposited on the endothelium of the cardiac graft microvasculature and proceed inflammatory responses, such as release of cytokines, infiltration of macrophages, increased vascular permeability, and microvascular thrombosis, which results in cardiac graft dysfunction [2, 3].

The presence of circulating DSAs in HTx negatively impacts clinical outcome after HTx. Due to different clinical implications, DSA can be divided into preformed and de novo DSA by the time detected. Preformed antibodies can reduce the possibility to obtain a compatible donor heart and may increase the risk of AMR after HTx. With regard to post-HTx setting, considerable evidences about the impacts of DSAs on outcomes such as rejection, cardiac allograft vasculopathy, and survival have been reported [2–4, 9].

4.1 Currently used methods to assess anti-HLA antibodies

There are several anti-HLA antibody screening methods, each with varying sensitivities, specificities, and clinical usefulness [5–7].

4.1.1 Crossmatching

4.1.1.1 Complement-dependent cytotoxicity (CDC) test

Patel and Terasaki reported a significant correlation between a positive CDC crossmatch (or lymphocyte cytotoxicity test methods) and hyperacute and accelerated acute kidney graft dysfunction in 1969 [5]. Recipient serum is mixed with T and B lymphocytes from the donor and complement source is added. A cytotoxic reaction suggests the presence of complement fixing DSAs. The advantage of the test is its high positive predictive value for HAR or early acute AMR, making it well-defined that a patient should not undergo transplant with a particular donor. The disadvantage of this test is that it requires donor leukocytes and recipient serum prior to transplantation and that it is based on in vitro complement-mediated lysis which may not be of physiological relevance. This method using T lymphocytes has been used for prospective crossmatching in Japan to select the recipient in heart, lung, pancreas, and kidney transplantation. And that using B-lymphocytes is used for reference crossmatching to select the recipient transplanted with these organs according to each transplant center protocol [6, 9].

4.1.1.2 Flow cytometry crossmatching

Flow cytometry crossmatching method consists of reacting recipient serum with donor lymphocytes and adding a fluorescent-labeled anti-human immunoglobulin secondary antibody [7, 8]. The shifts in the distribution of fluorescence signals are detected in this assay. In flow cytometric crossmatching, complement sources are not added. As this assay is more sensitive at detecting physiological reactions than CDC, this assay is widely used for crossmatching in many countries in solid organ transplant. However, not all DSAs determined by this method are cytotoxic to the cardiac graft because this assay cannot evaluate complement fixation ability of DSAs [7, 8]. The false positivity of this method may decrease the likelihood of obtaining a compatible donor heart. Therefore, due to extremely more severe organ shortage in Japan than other developed countries, flow cytometric crossmatching is used only as a reference to select the heart recipient to increase a chance to obtain a compatible donor heart [9].

4.1.1.3 Virtual crossmatching

The virtual crossmatch protocol was introduced on October 2006 at Texas Transplant Institute for all sensitized patients waiting for deceased donor kidney transplantation [33]. Briefly, HLA typing antibody screening is performed using flow PRA screen beads (One Lambda) for the presence or absence of HLA class I and II antibodies. HLA class I and II single antigens (SA) include A, B, and Cw loci and DR, DQ, DRw, and DP loci, respectively. All final crossmatches are carried out by flow cytometry.

The rationale for recommending virtual crossmatching is double staged: (1) use methods having the sensitivity of DSA detecting assay nearly equal to the CDC crossmatch test and (2) reduce the time and cost for choosing a compatible deceased donor by no longer performing prospective CDC crossmatch test. By undoing prospective CDC crossmatch test, the average turnaround time is reduced by 3 hours which allows quicker organ allocation with reasonable assurance that the sensitized patients at the top waiting list will have an adequate deceased donor with negative final crossmatch [33].

4.1.2 Screening for the presence or absence of DSAs

4.1.2.1 CDC panel reactive antibody screening

The method to detect the anti-HLA antibodies had historically been the CDC assay [5]. The sera were analyzed using a manufactured frozen lymphocyte panels, which consist of mononucleated cells isolated from 60 or 72 healthy individuals of known HLA typing of A and B locus antigens [34]. However, as these CDC PRA cell panel are currently less available, and its technique is more complicated than flow PRA screening, more sensitive assays shown below are widely used. However, CDC PRA remains an alternative to define the level of patient desensitization, in cross-matching with a specific donor to avoid HAR [4, 9].

4.1.2.2 Flow PRA screening

Flow PRA screening uses panels of beads coated with the equivalent of whole cell's HLA class 1 or 2 [35]. Often used for initial screening, it gives a qualitative result on an incomplete panel. Luminex PRA uses panels of beads also coated with the equivalent of whole cell's HLA class 1 or 2. PRAs are more sensitive than CDC but less sensitive than SAB assay. These PRA methods require expert interpretation and there is a possibility to miss antibodies [9].

4.1.2.3 Single antigen Luminex bead assay

SAB assay uses microbeads coated with unique HLA antigen/allele on each bead [35] and detects a specific anti-HLA IgG antibody using a single HLA antigen/allele being interested. SAB assays are the most sensitive, specific, and definitive of the bead assays, but are often considered overreactive, with ambiguous clinical significance. SAB assays are now commonly applied for determining specificities and quantities of antibodies against antigen of interest. SAB assay for preformed HLA antibodies is useful as a reference to establish the protocol of desensitization strategies before and at the time of HTx, to select an adequate compatible donor heart, and to decide posttransplant immunosuppressive regimen [4, 9, 18].

4.2 Complement binding antibodies

Since complement activation plays a major role in antibody-mediated immune response on transplanted graft, detection of ability of antibodies to bind specific complement components seems to provide further clinical benefit for the diagnosis of AMR. Conventional solid-phase assays, such as SAB assay, cannot distinguish between complement binding and non-complement binding antibodies, and the intensity of antibodies by mean fluorescence intensity (MFI) may not be the best index of cytotoxic ability of antibodies because not all antibodies with high MFI may be prejudicial to graft function [9, 36]. Detection of antibodies capable of binding the component of classical pathway, such as C1q, C4d, or C3d, may indicate the potential for antibody-mediated cell injury. The complement binding antibody assay may be potentially more specific than conventional solid-phase assays to predict immune response to donor antigen and more sensitive than CDC assay. Although the diagnostic approach using complement binding DSAs seems to be supportive for the more adequate donor matching with sensitized recipients than the CDC assay or other conventional indirect methods such as SAB assay, the usefulness of complement-fixing DSA assay for desensitization or posttransplant monitoring in HTx remains unclear.

4.2.1 Cascade of complement activation

Complemental cascade is a multifunctional system of receptors and regulators as well as effector molecules [37]. The classical complement pathway can be initiated by the binding of antigen–antibody complexes to the C1q protein. The binding of C1q changes conformation and activates serine protease C1r which then cleaves and activates the serine protease C1s. The activated C1s cleaves C4, yielding C4a and C4b, and C2, yielding C2a and C2b. The larger fragments C4b and C2a generate the classical pathway C3 convertase. This convertase then cleaves C3 into a small C3a fragment and a larger C3b fragment. While the anaphylatoxin C3a interacts with its C3a receptor to recruit leukocytes, C3b contributes to further downstream complement activation. A larger C3b binds to the cell surface. C4b can be regulated by decay accelerating factor dissociating C4b and C2a. Successful regulation of C4 by factor 1 leaves C4d as an end product that truncates the complement cascade. C3b is more versatile than C4b. Factor I also can cleave C3b to ultimately produce C3d, which is a ligand for complement receptor type 2 on B lymphocytes. Moreover, C3b can generate an alternative C3 convertase with factor B, which allows C3b to start an amplification loop that can greatly increase the amount of C3b deposited on a cell surface. Finally, C3b binds to the C3 convertase, to generate C5 convertase, which cleaves C5 into C5a and C5b. Subsequent interactions between C5b and other terminal components C6, C7, C8, and C9 generate the membrane attack complex (MAC) or the C5b-9 complex which makes pores on the target cell membranes to lysing (**Figure 1**).

4.2.2 Principles of C1q, C3d, and C4d binding assays

The C1q binding SAB (C1q SAB) assay (One Lambda, Canoga, USA) aims at defining HLA antibodies capable to bind C1q. Serum samples are first heat-inactivated to eliminate interference of endogenous complement components. Sera are incubated together with recombinant C1q. An antibody capable to bind C1q is detected by a phycoerythrin (PE)-conjugated anti-C1q antibody (**Figure 2**) [38]. As IgM or IgG cannot be identified by this anti-C1q antibody, C1q binding anti-HLA antibodies detected can be either IgM or IgG isotype.

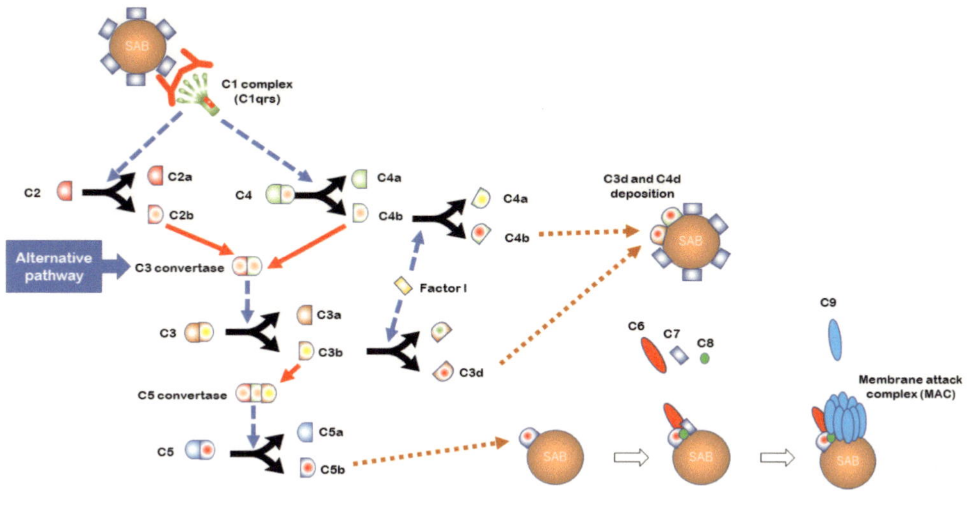

Figure 1.
Complement of classical complement pathway.

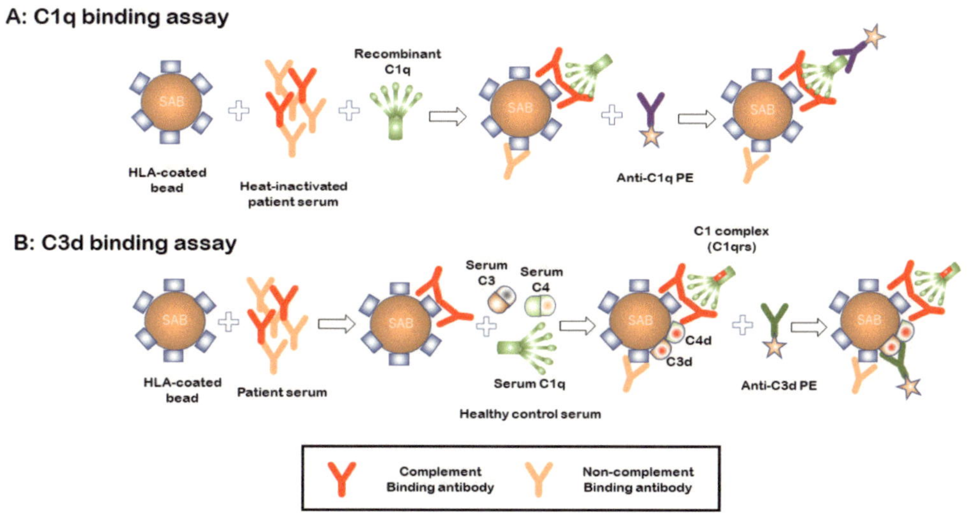

Figure 2.
Principles of C1q and C3d binding assays. (A) C1q binding assay: Heat-inactivated patient serum is incubated with single antigen beads (SABs) and recombinant C1q. Following a wash step, phycoerythrin-conjugated anti-C1q antibody is added to detect C1q binding HLA antibodies. (B) C3d binding assay: Patient serum is first incubated with SABs. Following binding of HLA antibodies to the beads, a healthy control serum as the complement source is added for further incubation. Following a wash step, PE conjugated anti-C3d antibody is added to detect C3d deposition on the beads.

Whereas C1q binding to antigen-bound antibody is the first step in activating classical complement pathway, binding of C1q to antibodies does not necessarily mean that all downstream events in this cascade will occur, as has been shown for human monoclonal HLA antibodies [39]. In this regard, C3d and C4d binding assays might be a more accurate modality to predict in vivo complement activation causing cell injury. As C1q binding to antibody triggers complement cascade once and then complement split products, such as C3d are clustered on beads in turn, the C3d assay may have a higher sensitivity than the C1q assay [40, 41]. As schematized in **Figure 2**, the C3d assay is like the C1q assay in methodology but does not need a recombinant complement product. Following an initial incubation of serum samples with SABs, healthy control human serum is added as a source of complement, and then an anti-human C3d detection antibody is added.

4.3 Significance of anti-HLA antibodies before and after HTx

4.3.1 Preformed anti-HLA antibody (anti-HLA antibody made before HTx)

Clinical significance of pretransplant sensitization and current modality to detect preformed DSAs are already described above. In summary, as non-CDC crossmatching are more sensitive for detecting DSAs than CDC assay, flow cytometry crossmatching or virtual crossmatching is more prevalent in the world. However, in patients negative for CDC crossmatching, positive for flow cytometry crossmatching is not associated with higher incidence or severity of cardiac graft failure than negative for flow cytometry crossmatching. Its high sensitivity for DSA detection may result in increasing of false positive for predicting HAR or early acute AMR and decreasing the opportunity of sensitized candidates to obtain a compatible donor heart especially in Japan where donor shortage is extremely severe [6]. Therefore, more precise sensitive tests should be added to CDC-based strategies to avoid the false positive. In recent years, there has been a great interest in the detection of DSAs with complement binding capacity to overcome these issues.

4.3.2 Donor-specific anti-HLA antibodies posttransplant

The development of anti-DSAs after HTx has been implicated in allograft injury. DSAs which are produced by sensitization after transplantation are called de novo DSA. Both preformed and de novo DSAs should be assessed for monitoring the efficacy of desensitization therapy and posttransplant immunosuppressive regimen. Solid-phase assays, such as the SAB assay, are recommended to detect circulating antibodies. A percent of PRA greater than 10% or preformed DSAs at the time of HTx increases the risk for suboptimal post-HTx outcome. Monitoring for DSAs should be performed at 1, 3, 6, and 12 months post-HTx in accordance with ISHLT guidelines [18]. Patients at low risk should be monitored annually, and sensitized patients should be monitored more frequently. In any patient with symptoms or signs of graft dysfunction, DSA testing should be performed. The presence of DSA with graft dysfunction including restrictive physiology should be considered for AMR treatment.

4.4 Clinical significance of complement binding antibody in AMR

Although DSAs can induce a wide spectrum of graft injuries from no damage to severe myocardial or endothelial injury, not all DSAs are responsible for causing AMR or the poor prognosis post-HTx [41–43]. Since improved analysis is needed to better distinguish DSAs relevant to clinical outcome, SAB assays for detecting complement binding capability of HLA antibodies (C1q, C3d) have been introduced [43–46] with the hypothesis that complement binding antibodies induce more severe graft injury than their non-activating counterparts [41]. Several studies have revealed significant association of C1q or C3d binding DSAs with high incidence of AMR or poor graft or patient survival [44, 45]. Although several studies have compared two complement binding assays, the superiority or difference of these diagnostic utilities remains unclear. Therefore, C1q or C3d binding DSA assay cannot be a definitive method to detect DSAs relevant to AMR. However, these assays can be a supportive method to decide immunotherapy.

4.4.1 Clinical applications of C1q biding assay for preformed DSA

Over the past two decades, sensitization rates in adult HTX candidates (PRA > 10%) have doubled from 7.7 to 13.5% [1]. An increased incidence is expected due to the increased application of left ventricular assist devices (LVADs) as a bridge to HTx strategy, improved congenital heart disease surgery with patients surviving to require HTx, and increased re-HTx. Although development of desensitization strategies is needed to enable successful HTx in these highly sensitized patients, LVAD infections remain the most frequent complication of LVAD care with high morbidity and mortality, and desensitization method should not be over-immunosuppressive. Therefore, clinical tools to evaluate DSAs relevant to desensitization efficacy are more required in HTx than in other solid organ transplantations.

In our institute, we have used C1q SAB assay as an auxiliary method to evaluate the effects of desensitization therapy.

4.4.1.1 Case

A 43-year-old gentleman with dilated cardiomyopathy who had been supported by a NIPRO extracorporeal LVAD (NIPRO Corp, Osaka, Japan) for 1677 days underwent HTx. As he had received a transfusion of packed red blood cells and platelets at the time of LVAD implantation and packed red blood cells for gastrointestinal bleedings several times, he had high intensity anti-HLA antibodies and had not been selected as a recipient of several donor hearts due to positive CRC crossmatching against the particular donor T lymphocytes. Therefore IVIg (5 g/day) was given for 5 days for desensitization treatment. The antibody level of eight anti-HLA antibodies was higher than 15,000 MFI assessed by SAB assay before IVIG treatment. However, in seven of those antibodies, the antibody level assessed by C1q SAB assay was lower than that assessed by SAB assay. Although the antibody levels of anti-HLA antibodies assessed by SAB assay 1 month after IVIG treatment were higher than those before IVIG treatment, the antibody levels of all the anti-HLA antibodies assessed by C1q SAB assay 1 month after IVIG treatment were lower than those before IVIG treatment (**Figure 3**).

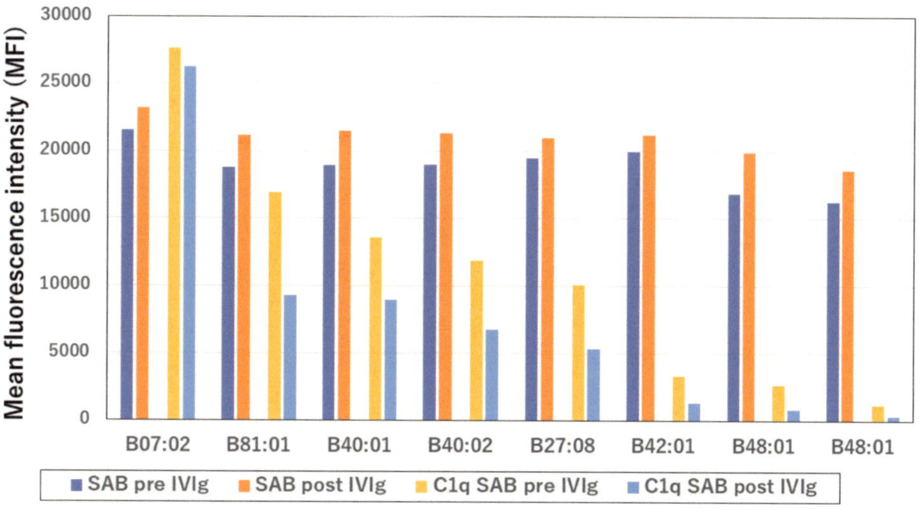

Figure 3.
Changes in mean fluorescence intensity by single antigen Luminex bead assay and C1q binding SAB assay before and 1 month after desensitization treatment. SAB, single antigen Luminex bead assay; C1q SAB, C1q binding SAB assay; IVIg, intravenous immune globulin.

After three courses of IVIg desensitization, he underwent HTx with a donor heart with negative prospective CDC crossmatching using the donor T lymphocytes. Although virtual SAB crossmatch showed preformed DSAs against HLA loci A2, A26, B35, and B65 with high MFI (**Table 1**), C1q SAB revealed that C1q binding abilities of these antibodies were all negative. Then we decided not to perform plasmapheresis or antithymocyte globulin in order to avoid over-immunosuppression. 20 mg of basiliximab was given IV just after discontinuing cardiopulmonary bypass and confirming hemostasis and at the 4th postoperative day. Maintenance immunosuppressive regimen consisted of Tac, MMF, and CS. Although routine EMB revealed pAMR 1 at 1 week after HTx, he experienced no hemodynamic compromise or cardiac graft dysfunction, and EMB revealed no further AMR or acute cellular rejection. He is currently at home with good cardiac graft function 2.5 years after HTx (**Table 2**).

4.4.2 Clinical application of C1q binding assay for maintenance immunosuppressive strategies

It is also known that not all patients with persistent production of DSA suffer loss of their allografts, indicating that DSAs are not equal in terms of their detrimental effects on allograft function. A C1q-positive de novo DSA has been reported to be associated with an increased rate of AMR and transplant glomerulopathy in kidney transplantation [46–49]. However, the prevalence and clinical significance of DSA characterized by C1q binding have not been well investigated in adult HTx patients [50–52].

In our clinical experience of 64 consecutive patients who received a HTx between May 1999 and January 2015, 12 patients had DSAs after HTx, but none had C1q binding antibodies. There were no significant differences in overall or cardiac event-free patient survival between DSA positive and negative patients with the same immunosuppressive regimen post-HTx (**Figure 4**). These data suggested that no reinforcement immunosuppressive regimen is needed, if the patient had no C1q binding DSA midterm after HTx [53].

			A		B		Cw	
HLA class I		**Recipient**	**33**	**—**	**44**	**—**	**14**	**—**
		Donor	**2**	**26**	**35**	**62**	**1**	**9**
DSA (MFI)	Pre-IVIG	SAB assay	11,429	57.3	13,725	13,911	90.4	397
		C1q SAB assay	0	0	0	0	1.35	0
	At HTx	SAB assay	3911	10.7	4629	7631	72.7	77.4
		C1q SAB assay	3.7	0	0	6.4	1.2	0.9
	2 months after HTx	SAB assay	315	37.9	633	3025	1300	12.1
		C1q SAB assay	0	0	0	0	0	0

HLA, human leukocyte antigen; DSA, donor-specific anti-HLA antibody; MFI, mean fluorescent intensity; SAB, single antigen Luminex bead assay; C1q SAB, C1q binding SAB assay; IVIg, intravenous immune globulin.

Table 2.
Human leukocyte antigen class I of the recipient and the donor and the antibody level of the donor-specific HLA antibodies assessed by single antigen Luminex bead assay and C1q binding SAB assay before IVIG therapy, at the time of heart transplantation and 2 months after heart transplantation.

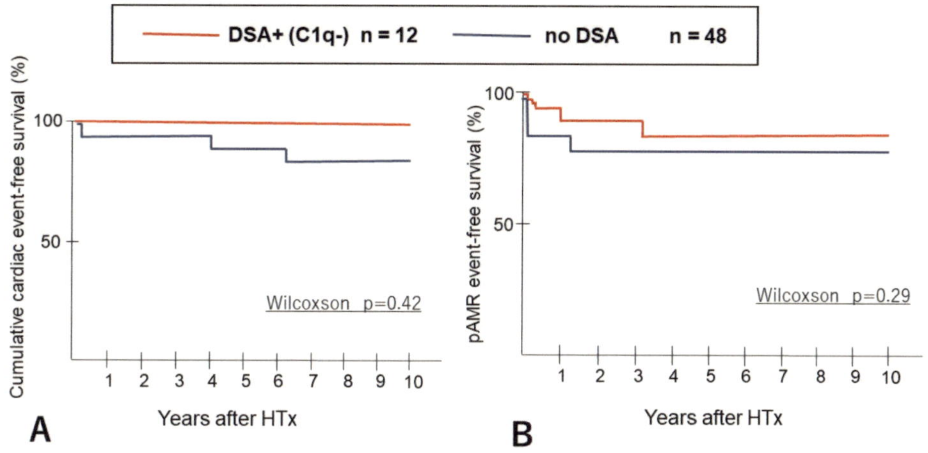

Figure 4.
Cumulative overall (A) and cardiac event-free (B) survival in patients with and without developing DSA. DSA, donor-specific anti-human leukocyte antigen; HTx, heart transplantation.

5. Conclusion

Over the past decades, sensitization rates in adult HTX candidates have doubled patients due to the expanding application of LVAD and prolonged waiting period. Sensitized HTx candidates have extended the waiting times for obtaining a compatible donor heart and increased mortality while waiting. An effective desensitization strategy has the potential to increase access to and success of HTx in sensitized patients, thus improving outcomes for this disadvantaged and growing transplant population. Although CDC PRA screening remains a standard method to define the efficacy of desensitization therapy, CDC PRA cell panels are currently less available, and its technique is complicated. Therefore, more sensitive assays flow PRA screening or SAB are widely used. However, flow cytometry is too sensitive to select the recipient, because not all DSAs determined by this method are cytotoxic to the cardiac graft. Although C1q or C3d binding DSA assay cannot be a definitive method to detect DSAs relevant to AMR, these assays can be a novel supportive method to decide immunotherapy.

Conflict of interest

None.

Author details

Takuya Watanabe and Norihide Fukushima*
Department of Transplant Medicine, National Cerebral and Cardiovascular Center, Suita, Osaka, Japan

*Address all correspondence to: nori@ncvc.go.jp

References

[1] Lund LH, Edwards LB, Kucheryavaya AY, Benden C, Dipchand AI, Goldfarb S, et al. The registry of the International Society for Heart and Lung Transplantation: Thirty-second official adult heart transplantation report—2015; focus theme: Early graft failure. The Journal of Heart and Lung Transplantation. 2015;**34**(10):1244-1254

[2] Colvin MM, Cook JL, Chang P, Francis G, Hsu DT, Kiernan MS, et al. Antibody-mediated rejection in cardiac transplantation: Emerging knowledge in diagnosis and management: A scientific statement from the American Heart Association. Circulation. 2015;**131**(18):1608-1639

[3] Berry GJ, Burke MM, Andersen C, Bruneval P, Fedrigo M, Fishbein MC, et al. The 2013 International Society for Heart and Lung Transplantation working formulation for the standardization of nomenclature in the pathologic diagnosis of antibody-mediated rejection in heart transplantation. The Journal of Heart and Lung Transplantation. 2013;**32**(12):1147-1162

[4] Kobashigawa J, Colvin M, Potena L, Dragun D, Crespo-Leiro MG, Delgado JF, et al. The management of antibodies in heart transplantation: An ISHLT consensus document. The Journal of Heart and Lung Transplantation. 2018;**37**(5):537-547

[5] Patel R, Terasaki PI. Significance of the positive crossmatch test in kidney transplantation. The New England Journal of Medicine. 1969;**280**(14):735-739

[6] Fukushima N, Ono M, Saiki Y, Sawa Y, Nunoda S, Isobe M. Registry report on heart transplantation in Japan (June 2016). Circulation Journal. 2017;**81**:298-303

[7] Scornik JC. Role of Flow Cytometry in Clinical Transplantation: Clinical Flow Cytometry. Williams and Wilkins; 1993. pp. 449-457

[8] Scornik JC. Detection of alloantibodies by flow cytometry: Relevance to clinical transplantation. Cytometry. 1995;**22**(4):259-263

[9] Kobashigawa J, Mehra M, West L, Kerman R, George J, Rose M, et al. Report from a consensus conference on the sensitized patient awaiting heart transplantation. The Journal of Heart and Lung Transplantation. 2009;**28**:213-225

[10] Brasile L, Zerbe T, Rabin B, Clarke J, Abrams A, Cerilli J. Identification of the antibody to vascular endothelial cells in patients undergoing cardiac transplantation. Transplantation. 1985;**40**:672-675

[11] Michaels P, Espejo M, Kobashigawa J, Alejos J, Burch C, Takemoto S, et al. Humoral rejection in cardiac transplantation: Risk factors, hemodynamic consequences and relationship to transplant coronary artery disease. The Journal of Heart and Lung Transplantation. 2003;**22**:58-69

[12] Kfoury A, Hammond M, Snow G, Stehlik J, Reid B, Long J, et al. Early screening for antibody-mediated rejection in heart transplant recipients. The Journal of Heart and Lung Transplantation. 2007;**26**:1264-1269

[13] Crespo-Leiro MG, Veiga-Barreiro A, Doménech N, Paniagua MJ, Piñon P, González-Cuesta M, et al. Humoral heart rejection (severe allograft dysfunction with no signs of cellular rejection or ischemia): Incidence, management, and the value of C4d for diagnosis. American Journal of Transplantation. 2005;**5**:2560-2564

[14] Hammond EH, Yowell RL, Nunoda S, Menlove RL, Renlund DG,

Bristow MR, et al. Vascular (humoral) rejection in heart transplantation: Pathologic observations and clinical implications. The Journal of Heart Transplantation. 1989;**8**:430-443

[15] Hathout E, Beeson WL, Kuhn M, Johnston J, Fitts J, Razzouk A, et al. Cardiac allograft vasculopathy in pediatric heart transplant recipients. Transplant International. 2006;**19**:184-189

[16] Loupy A, Cazes A, Guillemain R, Amrein C, Hedjoudje A, Tible M, et al. Very late heart transplant rejection is associated with microvascular injury, complement deposition and progression to cardiac allograft vasculopathy. American Journal of Transplantation. 2011;**11**:1478-1487

[17] Kfoury A, Hammond M, Snow G, Drakos S, Stehlik J, Fisher P, et al. Cardiovascular mortality among heart transplant recipients with asymptomatic antibody-mediated or stable mixed cellular and antibody-mediated rejection. The Journal of Heart and Lung Transplantation. 2009;**28**:781-784

[18] Costanzo MR, Dipchand A, Starling R, Anderson A, Chan M, Desai S, et al. The International Society of Heart and Lung Transplantation Guidelines for the care of heart transplant recipients. Journal of Heart and Lung Transplantation. 2010;**29**(8):914-956. DOI: 10.1016/j.healun.2010.05.034

[19] Weil R 3rd, Clarke DR, Iwaki Y, Porter KA, Koep LJ, Paton BC, et al. Hyperacute rejection of a transplanted human heart. Transplantation. 1981;**32**(1):71-72

[20] Saito S, Matsumiya G, Fukushima N, Sakaguchi T, Fujita T, Ueno T, et al. Successful treatment of cardiogenic shock caused by humoral cardiac allograft rejection. Circulation Journal. 2009;**73**(5):970-973

[21] Nwakanma LU, Williams JA, Weiss ES, Russell SD, Baumgartner WA, Conte JV. Influence of pretransplant panel-reactive antibody on outcomes in 8,160 heart transplant recipients in recent era. The Annals of Thoracic Surgery. 2007;**84**:1556-1563

[22] Chih S, Patel J. Desensitization strategies in adult heart transplantation—Will persistence pay off? Journal of Heart and Lung Transplantation. 2016;**35**:962-972

[23] Vo AA, Peng A, Toyoda M, Kahwaji J, Cao K, Lai CH, et al. Use of intravenous immune globulin and rituximab for desensitization of highly HLA-sensitized patients awaiting kidney transplantation. Transplantation. 2010;**89**:1095-1102

[24] Vo AA, Choi J, Cisneros K, Reinsmoen N, Haas M, Ge S, et al. Benefits of rituximab combined with intravenous immunoglobulin for desensitization in kidney transplant recipients. Transplantation. 2014;**98**:312-319

[25] Jordan SC, Tyan D, Stablein D, McIntosh M, Rose S, Vo A, et al. Evaluation of intravenous immunoglobulin as an agent to lower Allo sensitization and improve transplantation in highly sensitized adult patients with end-stage renal disease: Report of the NIH IG02 trial. Journal of the American Society of Nephrology. 2004;**15**:3256-3262

[26] Montgomery RA, Lonze BE, King KE, et al. Desensitization in HLA-in compatible kidney recipients and survival. The New England Journal of Medicine. 2011;**365**:318-326

[27] Dawson KL, Parulekar A, Seethamraju H. Treatment of hyperacute antibody-mediated lung allograft rejection with eculizumab. The Journal of Heart and Lung Transplantation. 2012;**31**(12):1325-1326

[28] Cornell LD, Schinstock CA, Gandhi MJ, Kremers WK, Stegall MD. Positive crossmatch kidney transplant recipients treated with eculizumab: Outcomes beyond 1 year. American Journal of Transplantation. 2015;**15**:1293-1302

[29] Patel J, Reinsmoen N, Kittleson M. Plasmapheresis and bortezomib for sensitized patients awaiting heart transplantation—Worth the effort? The Journal of Heart and Lung Transplantation. 2015;**34**(Suppl):S30-S31

[30] Patel J, Everly M, Chang D, Kittleson M, Reed E, Kobashigawa J. Reduction of alloantibodies via proteasome inhibition in cardiac transplantation. The Journal of Heart and Lung Transplantation. 2011;**30**:1320-1326

[31] Leech SH, Rubin S, Eisen HJ, et al. Cardiac transplantation across a positive prospective lymphocyte cross-match in sensitized recipients. Clinical Transplantation. 2003;**17**(Suppl 9):17-26

[32] Pisani BA, Mullen GM, Malinowska K, Lawless CE, Mendez J, Silver MA, et al. Plasmapheresis with intravenous immunoglobulin G is effective in patients with elevated panel reactive antibody prior to cardiac transplantation. The Journal of Heart and Lung Transplantation. 1999;**18**:701-706

[33] Zangwill SD, Ellis TM, Zlotocha J, Jaquiss RD, Tweddell JS, Mussatto KA, et al. The virtual crossmatch--a screening tool for sensitized pediatric heart transplant recipients. Pediatric Transplantation. 2006;**10**(1):38-41

[34] Available from: https://www.onelambda.com/en/products-services/products/antibody-.detection/lambda-cell-trayslct.html

[35] Cecka JM. Calculated PRA, (CPRA): The new measure of sensitization for transplant candidates. American Journal of Transplantation. 2010;**10**:26-29

[36] Cravedi P, Heeger PS. Complement as a multifaceted modulator of kidney transplant injury. The Journal of Clinical Investigation. 2014;**124**(6):2348-2354

[37] Nesargikar PN, Spiller B, Chavez R. The complement system: History, pathways, cascade and inhibitors. European Journal of Microbiology and Immunology. 2012;**2**:103-111. DOI: 10.1556/EuJMI.2.2012.2.2

[38] Karahan GE, Claas FHJ, Heidt S. Technical challenges and clinical relevance of single antigen bead C1q/C3d testing and IgG subclass analysis of human leukocyte antigen antibodies. Transplant International. 2018;**31**:1189-1197

[39] Duquesnoy RJ, Marrari M, Jelenik L, Zeevi A, Claas FH, Mulder A. Structural aspects of HLA class I epitopes reacting with human monoclonal antibodies in Ig-binding, C1q-binding and lymphocytotoxicity assays. Human Immunology. 2013;**74**:1271

[40] Lachmann PJ. The amplification loop of the complement pathways. Advances in Immunology. 2009;**104**:115

[41] Lan JH, Tinckam K. Clinical utility of complement dependent assays in kidney transplantation. Transplantation. 2018;**102**(1S Suppl 1): S14-S22

[42] Tyan DB. New approaches for detecting complement-fixing antibodies. Current Opinion in Organ Transplantation. 2012;**17**(4):409-415

[43] Min JW, Lee H, Choi BS, Park CW, Yang CW, Kim YS, et al. Clinical impact of pre-transplant antibodies against angiotensin II type I receptor and major histocompatibility complex class I-related chain a in kidney transplant patients. Annals of Laboratory

Medicine. 2018;**38**(5):450-457. DOI: 10.3343/alm.2018.38.5.450

[44] Sicard A, Ducreux S, Rabeyrin M, Couzi L, McGregor B, Badet L, et al. Detection of C3d-binding donor-specific anti-HLA antibodies at diagnosis of humoral rejection predicts renal graft loss. Journal of the American Society of Nephrology. 2015;**26**(2):457-467. DOI: 10.1681/ASN.2013101144

[45] Comoli P, Cioni M, Tagliamacco A, Quartuccio G, Innocente A, Fontana I, et al. Acquisition of C3d-binding activity by de novo donor-specific HLA antibodies correlates with graft loss in nonsensitized pediatric kidney recipients. American Journal of Transplantation. 2016;**16**(7):2106-2116. DOI: 10.1111/ajt.13700

[46] Kim JJ, Shaw O, Martin C, Michaelides G, Balasubramaniam R, Sebire NJ, et al. Clinical risk stratification of paediatric renal transplant recipients using C1q and C3d fixing of de novo donor-specific antibodies. Pediatric Nephrology. 2018;**33**(1):167-174. DOI: 10.1007/s00467-017-3772-7

[47] Chen G, Sequeira F, Tyan DB. Novel C1q assay reveals a clinically relevant subset of human leukocyte antigen antibodies independent of immunoglobulin G strength on single antigen beads. Human Immunology. 2011;**72**:849-858

[48] Crespo M, Torio A, Mas V, Redondo D, Pérez-Sáez MJ, Mir M, et al. Clinical relevance of pretransplant anti-HLA donor-specific antibodies: Does C1q-fixation matter? Transplantation Immunology. 2013;**29**:28-33

[49] Piazza A, Poggi E, Ozzella G, Adorno D. Post-transplant development of C1q-positive HLA antibodies and kidney graft survival. Clinical Transplantation. 2013:367-375. Available from: https://terasaki.org/store/CH44-Piazza

[50] Onwuemene OA, Heath DM, Hartman C, Wong ECC. Role of C1q complement fixing antibody assay in therapeutic plasma exchange management of pediatric cardiac antibody mediated rejection. Journal of Clinical Apheresis. 2017;**32**(4):279-281

[51] Das BB, Lacelle C, Zhang S, Gao A, Fixler D. Complement (C1q) binding de novo donor-specific antibodies and cardiac-allograft vasculopathy in pediatric heart transplant recipients. Transplantation. 2018;**102**(3):502-509

[52] Farrero Torres M, Pando MJ, Luo C, Luikart H, Valantine H, Khush K. The role of complement-fixing donor-specific antibodies identified by a C1q assay after heart transplantation. Clinical Transplantation. 2017;**31**(11):e13121. DOI: 10.1111/ctr.13121

[53] Sato T, Seguchi O, Yanase M, Kumai Y, Matsuda S, Kuroda K, et al. Clinical implication of non-complement-binding donor-specific anti-HLA antibodies in heart transplant recipients -risk stratification by C1q-binding capacity. Clinics in Surgery. 2017;**2**:1703

Chapter 4

Immunosuppression and Viral Infections

Seema Naik, Kevin Rakszawski, Joseph Cioccio, Hong Zheng and Hiroko Shike

Abstract

Immunosuppression is commonly used for prevention of graft rejection in solid organ transplantation (SOT) and prevention of graft versus host disease in hematopoietic allogeneic stem cell transplant (ASCT). In ASCT, immunosuppression is used to control GVHD and can be tapered off within 6–12 months after transplantation. SOT recipients require lifelong immunosuppression to prevent graft rejection, making them susceptible to serious viral infections including EBV PTLD. EBV PTLD occurs within the first 6 months following ASCT prior to effective reconstitution of cytotoxic T lymphocytes (CTL). Our understanding on EBV-related PTLD is mostly extrapolated from SOT-associated PTLD. Features of conditioning and use of serotherapy remain important in development of EBV PTLD. Other viral infections that occur early post-transplant include CMV, HHV6, BK, and adenovirus, and usually correspond to degree of immunosuppression post-transplant. These infections are associated with significant morbidity and mortality. However, the current literature lacks information on outcomes of viral infections related to immunosuppression. Alternative donor ASCT are now more common, and patients are more susceptible to multiple viral infectious complications at the peak of immunosuppression and require monitoring for viral infections in these immunosuppressed patients.

Keywords: immunosuppression, EBV PTLD, CMV, HSV, VZV, BK, HHV6

1. Immunosuppression

Immunosuppression is commonly used for prevention of graft rejection in solid organ transplantation (SOT) and prevention of graft versus host disease in hematopoietic allogeneic stem cell transplant (ASCT). In solid organ transplantation (SOT), the donor grafts are recognized as non-self by the recipient's immune system. The recipient immune system can cause T-cell-mediated rejection and antibody-mediated rejection at any time. Immunosuppression is critical to control the recipient immune system and protect donor organs from rejection. Therefore, immunosuppression is generally necessary as long as the patient retains a viable donor graft.

In allogenic hematopoietic cell transplantation, donor-derived hematopoietic stem cells and lymphocytes replace the hematopoietic system as well as the immune system of the recipient. While donor T-cells provide anti-pathogen and anti-tumor activity to the recipient, donor-derived alloreactive T-cells are responsible for graft versus host disease (GVHD). Immunosuppression is used to control acute and chronic GVHD. However, alloreactive T-cells are eventually eliminated in most patients, and immunosuppression can be tapered off within 6–12 months after transplantation in ASCT. Solid organ transplant recipients, on the other hand, require lifelong immunosuppression to prevent graft rejection, making them susceptible to EBV virus mediated post-transplant lymphoproliferative disorder (PTLD). In ASCT, some patients who develop chronic GVHD also need prolonged immunosuppression requiring monitoring and treatment of complications related to serious viral infections.

In cord transplant recipients and, more recently, in haploidentical transplant and mismatched transplant patients, with the effect of antithymocyte globulin (ATG) and other T-cell depleting regimens, patients are even more susceptible than usual to either single or multiple viral infectious complications at the peak of immunosuppression. Use of TNF receptor blockers including etanercept and infliximab for GVHD or Crohn disease, the use of other interleukin inhibitors for skin GVHD, and other autoimmune disorders are additional examples of ongoing immunosuppression that would require monitoring for viral infections and complications in these immunosuppressed patients.

The most common immunosuppression to prevent GVHD is the use of calcineurin inhibitors tacrolimus and cyclosporine. Calcineurin is an essential enzyme in the activation of T-cells. Both tacrolimus and cyclosporine have similar mechanisms of action and efficacy. In the post-transplant period, monitoring of tacrolimus and cyclosporine serum levels is performed as a surrogate for depth and degree of immunosuppression. In the early post-transplant period, a higher serum levels are essential until alloreactive T-cells are eliminated, at which point lower serum levels can still prevent GVHD. Other immunosuppressants used post-transplant include mycophenolate mofetil and mycophenolate sodium, which exhibit a cytostatic effect on T- and B-lymphocytes. Cyclophosphamide is now routinely given in the post haploidentical or mismatched transplant setting to reduce the incidence of GVHD by selective removal of alloreactive donor T-cells.

In the post-treatment phase beyond 100 days, the presence of chronic GVHD is the main determinant of infection. Patients who developed acute GVHD experience approximately 60% more infections than patients who do not develop acute GVHD. Furthermore, patients who experience chronic GVHD have their immunosuppression increased or restarted, therefore increasing the risk of infection.

2. EBV infection

EBV PTLD develops in approximately 1% of patients post ASCT. It is highly related to EBV reactivation. Risk factors that associate with high incidence of EBV-related PTLD include older age at transplant, T-cell depletion-containing conditioning regimens, antithymocyte globulin (ATG) use, and grafts derived from unrelated or HLA-mismatched donors [1–5]. PTLD in ASCT patients occurs in the younger age group, with shorter duration of onset as compared to (SOT) solid organ transplantation.

EBV PTLD occurs more commonly in pediatric patients than in adults because more pediatric patients are EBV naïve. PTLD can occur during the post-transplant period after both myeloablative and non-myeloablative ASCT. The degree and duration of immunosuppression plays a major role in the development of PTLD. Cytotoxic T lymphocytes (CTLs) provide a defense mechanism against EBV-infected B cells in immunocompetent individuals. However, T cell function is impaired post allogeneic transplant which leads to the development of PTLD. In vivo T cell depletion (TCD) with antithymocyte globulin (ATG) or alemtuzumab (AL) is commonly used in ASCT. As reduced intensity conditioning (RIC) and matched unrelated donor (MUD) transplants are now being performed more frequently, ATG and AL have become integral components of preparative regimens to facilitate engraftment and reduce the incidence and severity of GVHD. Delayed T cell reconstitution following T cell depletion accounts for infectious complications including PTLD, which is associated with increased mortality [3, 4].

EBV PTLD can occur later in the most severely immunocompromised patients with additional risk factors such as donor and recipient mismatch, graft manipulation with T cell depletion as well as the degree and duration of immunosuppression. Prevention of PTLD involves limiting the duration and degree of immunosuppression, while still maintaining the adequacy of the donor graft. Achieving a balance of reduction in immunosuppression and preventing graft rejection or graft versus host disease can be challenging. Antiviral prophylaxis may also play a role in preventing PTLD. The use of antiviral agents such as acyclovir, valganciclovir, and ganciclovir are common for HSV, CMV, and EBV prophylaxis, though data is very limited for prevention of EBV PTLD [2–5].

EBV monitoring of high-risk patient facilitates preemptive rituximab or tapering of immunosuppression upon viremia proceeding PTLD. Successful clearance of EBV and prevention of PTLD has been reported with B-cell depletion by rituximab [6–8]. On the other hand, antiviral agents, such as acyclovir, ganciclovir, and valganciclovir are not widely used for prevention, due to limited data. [2–5]. The use of "Off-the-shelf," third-party EBV-specific CTLs is a new promising approach to treat refractory PTLD to rituximab or immunosuppression tapering [3]. Treatment algorithm for EBV PTLD is as shown in **Tables 1** and 2.

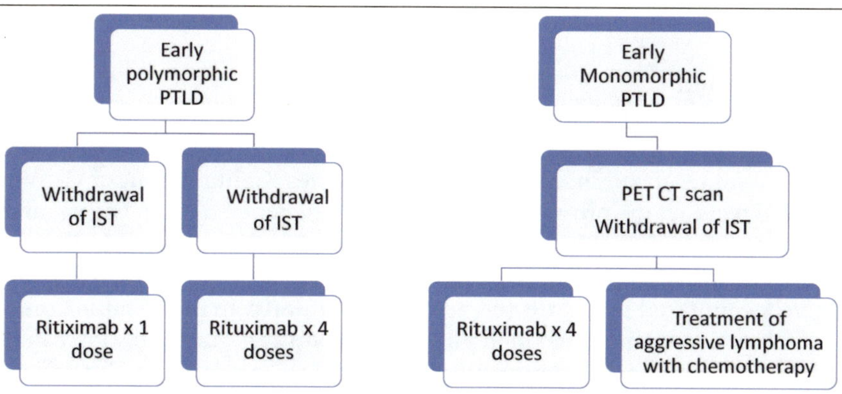

Table 1.
Treatment algorithm for EBV positive PTLD.

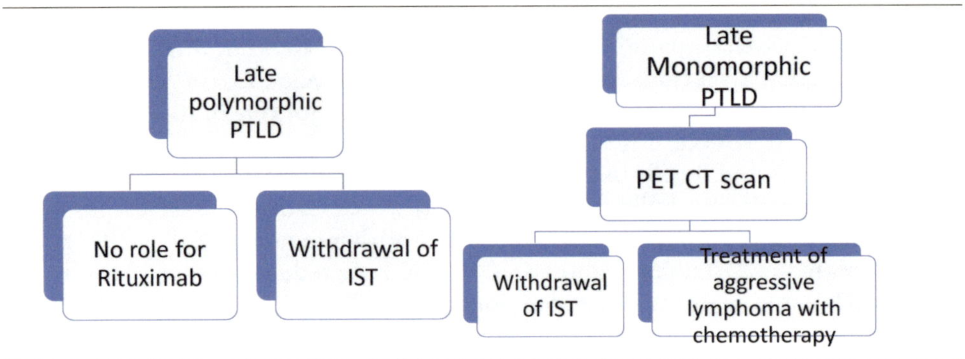

Table 2.
Treatment algorithm for EBV negative PTLD.

3. Other viral infections

Other viral infections that occur early post-transplant include CMV, HHV6, BK, and adenovirus, and usually correspond to degree of immunosuppression post-transplant [4, 9]. However, the current literature lacks information on outcomes of viral infections as well as the influence of graft sources, such as comparison of outcomes between umbilical cord blood transplant (UCBT) and haploidentical transplant (haplo) with post-transplant cyclophosphamide (PTCy) [10]. These infections usually occur within in early post-transplant period prior to effective immune reconstitution [1, 11, 12]. Despite advances in antiviral therapy, severe infections still remain a major cause of death after alternative donor ASCT [5, 9, 13].

In a prospective analysis of immune reconstitution in double UCBT recipients and matched unrelated donor (MUD) recipients, CD3 recovery was significantly delayed in the double UCBT group compared with MUD group for as long as 6 months after ASCT [5, 9, 13]. These unique properties of UCBT may contribute to a high risk of infection reported in some studies. Novel strategies are now being developed to combat viral infections including the virus-specific or trivirus-specific (adenovirus, Epstein-Barr virus, and cytomegalovirus) CTLs [14–16]. Early diagnostic information regarding viral infections is critically important in the current era of emerging new therapies for viral infections.

4. CMV infection

CMV infection occurs in 50–80% of the population and CMV virus is maintained in a latent reservoir in mononuclear leukocytes. Containment of CMV in its latent state affects a large proportion of host immune repertoire. In young adults, 1–2% of CD4 and CD8 T cells are CMV-reactive, which rise to up to 30–40% in the elderly. For the majority of CMV-infected individuals, asymptomatic reactivation is effectively countered by innate and adaptive immunity. In the immunocompromised ASCT patients, unconstrained viral replication and dissemination can lead to CMV disease, and increased mortality due to end-organ damage. The efficacy of conventional antiviral therapies including ganciclovir and foscarnet is limited in the setting CMV disease with end-organ involvement [17].

CMV-seropositive patients will experience CMV dissemination after ASCT, particularly in the context of transplant using T cell-depleted or matched unrelated donor (MUD) grafts. In CMV-seronegative patients, CMV infection is prevented through selection of CMV-seronegative grafts, but 20–40% of CMV-seronegative patients who receive CMV-seropositive grafts develop primary CMV infection. Untreated, 50% of ASCT patients with CMV reactivation will develop CMV disease. The current clinical practice uses close surveillance monitoring of CMV DNA burden by quantitative PCR (qPCR). Preemptive antiviral pharmacotherapy and prophylactic therapy strategies are used to reduce the incidence of CMV disease after ASCT. Novel antiviral pharmacotherapies including maribavir, letermovir, and brincidofovir are under clinical trial development but have not yet clearly demonstrated superiority or lesser toxicity compared to conventional antiviral agents [17].

5. Adenovirus viral infections

Adenovirus (AdV) infections are much more common in pediatric patients (20–26%) than in adults (9%) undergoing ASCT. In the severely immunocompromised patients, Adv can cause severe respiratory viral disease, hepatitis, and colitis. Other complications include hemorrhagic cystitis and adenoviral keratoconjunctivitis. AdV infection can cause subclinical viremia, viremia with disease symptoms, and disseminated disease. The incidence of disseminated disease is 1–7% with mortality of 8–26%. Rapidly increasing or persistent viremia is associated with the occurrence of severe adenoviral disease both in children and in adults. Monitoring of the viral load by blood AdV qPCR is far superior with high sensitivity. A study in adult ASCT recipients has reported an infection rate of 2.5% with pneumonia occurring in 24% of cases as the most common cause of death. Viral gastrointestinal shedding prior to transplant is found to be associated with increased risk of viremia after ASCT [18]. Treatment of adenoviral infections include Cidofovir, brincidofovir (compassionate use in children) and use of IVIG as well as taper of immunosuppression. More recent studies have used nucleofection to introduce DNA plasmids encoding multiple immunogenic antigens from CMV, EBV, and adenovirus into APCs to control lethal adenoviral infections.

6. HHV6 infection

Human herpesvirus 6 (HHV6), a member of β-herpesvirus subfamily, establishes primary infection as exanthem subitum in the normal pediatric population. With time, it establishes latency in $CD34^+$ cells, monocytes, and macrophages, similar to cytomegalovirus (CMV). Over the last decade, HHV6 has been increasingly recognized as an opportunistic and potentially life-threatening pathogen after ASCT [1–5, 9, 13–16, 18]. Following ASCT, HHV6 infections are caused by reactivation of the virus from latency. HHV6 reactivation is detected in the blood of 40–60% of patients after ASCT, most often by use of qPCR for viral-specific sequences.

HHV6 viremia has been reported in association with varying organ dysfunction and clinical syndromes including delayed/impaired platelet recovery, myelosuppression, encephalitis, fever, rash, hepatitis, pneumonitis, gastroduodenitis, CMV reactivation, and GVHD.

Treatment indications are uncertain in patients with HHV6 viremia following ASCT. HHV6 encephalitis is potentially fatal and is a common indication for treatment. Only one trial evaluated preemptive treatment of HHV6 based on a positive qPCR test. The development of reliable clinical guidelines for the management of

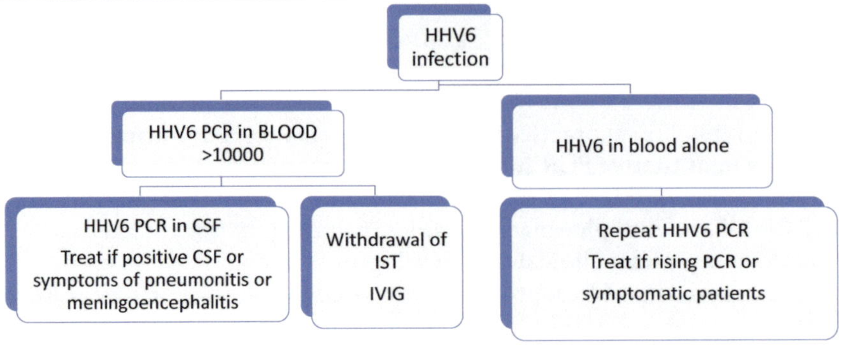

Table 3.
Treatment of HHV6 infection.

HHV6 viremia in ASCT recipients has historically been limited by the lack of specificity of viremia testing and by the lack of specific HHV6 clinical syndromes. It is also confounded by the occurrence of asymptomatic viremia, which often resolves without intervention. Treatment algorithm for HHV6 is as shown in **Table 3**.

7. BK virus infection

The BK virus infection is associated with hemorrhagic cystitis in ASCT recipients. Treatment interventions are mainly focused on supportive measures including hyperhydration, continuous bladder irrigation, and topical agents to alter the bladder mucosal lining. In the recent years, BK virus PCR in the urine and plasma has helped with early detection of BK virus infection and BK hemorrhagic cystitis (BK-HC) as higher urine and plasma viral loads are associated with disease manifestation including BK-HC [19, 20].

Other treatments of BK-HC aim at repair and regeneration of the urothelial mucosa through hyperbaric oxygen therapy or by topical application of fibrin. Use of hyperbaric oxygen has limited availability and also the risk of barotrauma and claustrophobia [19]. Finally, topical fibrin glue applications to the damaged bladder mucosa to achieve hemostasis through cystoscopy have been reported in single-center retrospective series of 35 patients with complete response rate of 83%. Several compounds to reduce bleeding have been used in small studies which include FXIII concentrate, intravesical sodium hyaluronate, estrogens or choreito extract granules with response rates between 50 and 100% [19]. Brincidofovir, a lipid conjugate of cidofovir has a potent and long-lasting inhibitory effect on BK virus replication in vitro studies but no data are available on the clinical use in BK nephropathy after ASCT. Brincidofovir may have the future indication for symptomatic BK-HC considering the absence of alternative antivirals with a better safety and tolerability profile [19, 20].

The reduction of immunosuppression has been used successfully in kidney transplant patients to prevent and/or treat BK nephropathy, but there is no evidence that it has a favorable risk/benefit ratio in ASCT patients due to the risk of worsening donor alloreactivity and severity of GVHD. Unlike for BK nephropathy, there is no documented benefit in using intravenous immunoglobulin (IVIG) for BK-HC. Extrapolating from use in BK virus nephropathy in renal transplant patients, cidofovir and leflunomide are only currently available agents for the treatment of BK-HC and fluoroquinolone antibiotics are considered as possible prophylactic agents.

Treatment algorithm for BK is as shown **Table 4**.

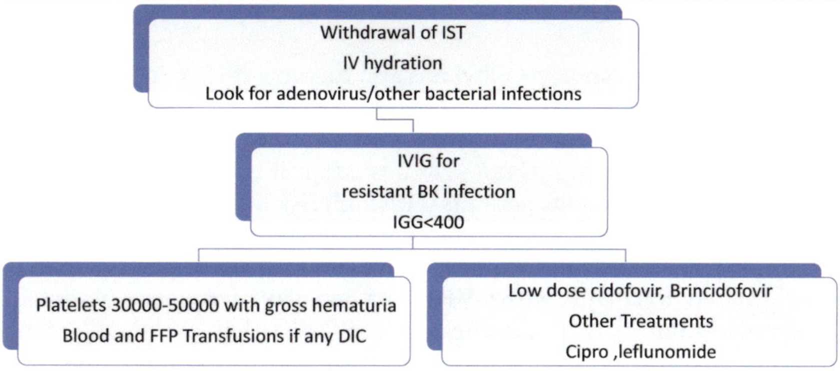

Table 4.
Treatment of BK infection /BK cystitis.

8. HSV/VZV infection: herpesviruses

The herpesvirus group currently consists of eight members, six of which have been implicated as important pathogens in ASCT recipients. During recent years, antiviral agents are used both for prevention and therapy in ASCT patients. Currently available anti-herpesvirus drugs are acyclovir and its prodrug valacyclovir, penciclovir and its prodrug famciclovir, ganciclovir with the prodrug valganciclovir, cidofovir, and foscarnet. All of the available drugs, except foscarnet, are nucleoside analogues and require phosphorylation by viral or cellular enzymes to become activated (**Tables 5** and **6**).

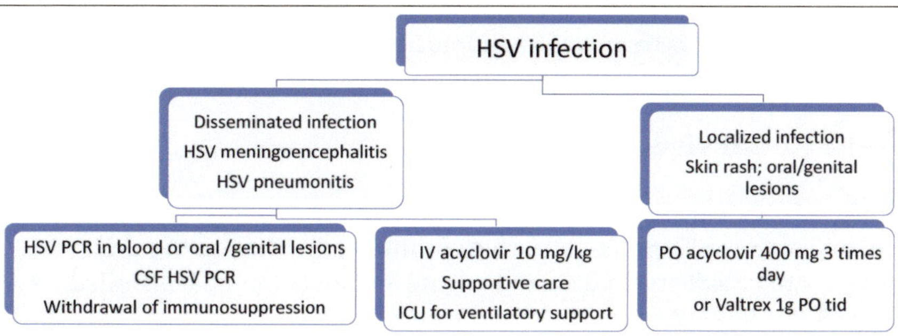

Table 5.
Treatment of HSV infection.

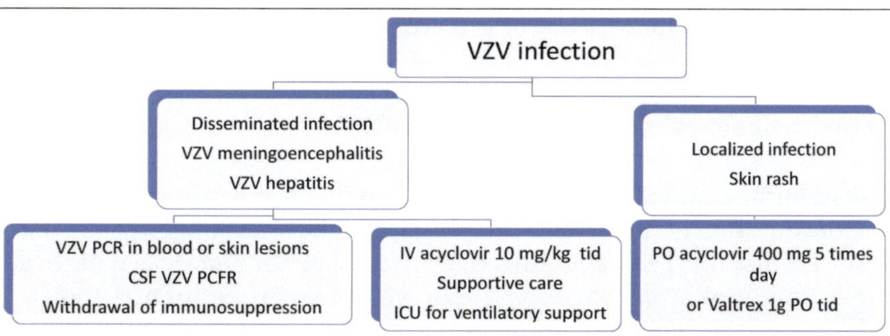

Table 6.
Treatment of VZV infection.

9. Herpes simplex virus (HSV)

The first controlled studies of prophylaxis and therapy of HSV in ASCT patients were performed more than 20 years ago, showing that effective antiviral agents can make an important impact on morbidity and mortality. The results from these early trials showed that acyclovir prophylaxis is indicated in all HSV-seropositive ASCT recipients and in some autologous patients with high risk for mucositis [21]. The duration of antiviral prophylaxis should be adjusted for each individual but should be continued throughout the aplastic phase. A longer duration of prophylaxis should be considered in patients with GVHD or a history of frequent reactivations before transplantation [21]. It is important to realize that HSV reactivations frequently occur quickly after prophylaxis is stopped and might require therapy long-term prophylaxis [22].

Valacyclovir, the prodrug of acyclovir, is also used as prophylaxis but no controlled studies have been performed in transplant patients. Valacyclovir gives similar acyclovir serum levels to IV acyclovir in neutropenic patients. Established HSV disease can be treated either orally or intravenously. The most commonly used drug is acyclovir, which should be given intravenously in patients with disseminated HSV or suspected central nervous system (CNS) disease therapy [22].

The most frequently used agents for HSV prophylaxis and therapy all require the viral enzyme thymidine kinase for activation. Virus resistance occurs with the development of mutant lacking this enzyme. Although acyclovir has been in use for almost 20 years, there has been only a moderate increase in acyclovir-resistant strains of HSV. Recently, acyclovir-resistant HSV have become more common, in unrelated and HLA-mismatched ASCT recipients and in patients who develop GVHD. The recommended drug for acyclovir-resistant HSV has been foscarnet. Currently, the only available antiviral drug available for treatment of double resistant HSV is cidofovir. However, although sensitive *in vitro*, the clinical response in high-risk ASCT patients treated with cidofovir has been variable [22].

10. Varicella-Zoster virus (VZV)

VZV infection is a very severe complication in ASCT patients. The risk is highest in children due to the epidemiologic pattern of infection. The live Varicella vaccine has been shown to be safe in children with acute leukemia but no controlled trial in ASCT recipients has been published and its use is not recommended earlier than 24 months after transplantation. Varicella-zoster immune globulin is the recommended prophylactic measure in seronegative ASCT recipients after an exposure to varicella has occurred if it can be given within 4 days of exposure [21, 22]. Another option is antiviral chemoprophylaxis with acyclovir or valacyclovir but there is no published data regarding the efficacy of this strategy.

11. Prevention of reactivated infection of VZV

The risk of herpes zoster is highest between 3 and 6 months after transplantation. Thus, the duration of antiviral prophylaxis must be long enough to prevent reactivated VZV disease. Two randomized, controlled studies have been performed comparing 6 months of prophylactic acyclovir with place. In addition, a non-controlled study of acyclovir or ganciclovir prophylaxis was recently published. All three studies showed that acyclovir was effective in reducing the risk for herpes zoster during the 6 months of therapy but at 12 months after transplantation there was no longer any difference. An unpublished study by Bowden and colleagues from the Seattle group indicated that the rebound in VZV disease does not occur if the prophylaxis is prolonged to 12 months [23]. Valacyclovir has not been studied for VZV prophylaxis, but the rate of VZV disease was reduced in a study when valacyclovir was compared to acyclovir as CMV prophylaxis. Some centers, however, do use valacyclovir as long-term prophylaxis against VZV [21, 22].

12. Treatment of VZV disease

The recommended therapy for a primary varicella or disseminated herpes zoster is intravenous acyclovir 10 mg/kg (or 500 mg/m^2) three times daily. For localized dermatomal herpes zoster, oral acyclovir 800 mg given five times daily was compared with IV acyclovir in a small randomized study in ASCT patients and the outcome was comparable. Famciclovir 500 mg given three times daily was compared with acyclovir 800 mg five times daily in ASCT, solid organ transplant and oncology patients, and the results indicated similar efficacy. No controlled study has been performed with valacyclovir given for treatment of a herpes zoster in ASCT patients. VZV resistance to acyclovir is rare but has been reported after ASCT [22, 23].

Treatment algorithm for HSV/VZV is as shown in **Tables 5** and **6**.

13. Other upper respiratory infections

The conditioning regimen has an impact on the incidence of these infections. Even though the patients with myeloablative and non-myeloablative conditioning have similar incidences for respiratory viral infections, LRI are significantly increased during the early post myeloablative ASCT period compared to non-myeloablative ASCT [14, 15].

14. Treatment of respiratory viral infections post ASCT

Lower overall survival seen with respiratory virus infection is due to bacterial co-infection causing increased mortality in high-risk patients with lymphopenia, CMV DNAemia at the time of viral LRI and need for oxygen support. Over the past years, more respiratory infections in ASCT recipients have been reported due to the use of new multiplex polymerase chain reaction (PCR) tests with higher sensitivity, specificity compared to conventional viral culture and antibody assays. Early diagnosis and treatment are important to improve outcomes of patients with upper respiratory viral infections (URI) s and lower respiratory viral infections (LRI)s [14, 15].

15. CMV-specific T cell lines and multi virus-specific T cell lines (multi-VST)

Immunotherapeutic strategies to hasten T cell recovery after ASCT remain an option as an adjunct to drug treatments. CMV-seropositive patients who are recipients of T cell-depleted CMV-seronegative donor or cord blood grafts are at highest risk from CMV-associated morbidity and mortality. Severe GVHD and drug-induced T cell dysfunction are also risk factors for CMV-related morbidity.

Recovery of CMV-specific CD4 responses is critical to effective antiviral responses, and restoration of both antigen-specific CD4 and CD8 T cell populations to control CMV is critical in this scenario [14–16].

An alternative to CMV-specific T cell clones is the use of CMV-specific T cell lines. In a clinical study, a single infusion of CMV-specific CD4 T cells showed plasma CMV clearance in 63% of patients. The HLA-A2–restricted pp65 peptide NLVPMVATV (NLV) is also being used but a major disadvantage of the HLA-A2–restricted NLV peptide approach is the restriction of benefit to HLA-A2^{+} patients only [10, 16, 17].

Multi-VST lines represent an interesting option to target multiple viral infections using adoptive cell therapy. Such lines can be manufactured either with APC systems using overlapping peptide pools from multiple viruses, or with other gene transfer approaches by the use of an adenoviral vector encoding the CMV-associated pp65 antigen to transduce APCs (MoDCs and EBV-transformed lymphoblastoid cell lines [LCLs]) before coculture with PBMCs or naive cord blood. This method delivers both MHC class I-dependent processing and expansion of CMV-reactive CD8 T cells, and MHC class II-dependent processing and presentation of adenovirus/EBV/CMV-associated peptides to drive expansion of virus-specific CD4 T cells. The adenoviral transfer vector promotes anti-adenoviral T cell specificity (bispecific CTLs), and if EBV-transformed B cells are used in lieu of MoDCs, then additional EBV-specificity is generated (trispecific CTLs) [10, 16, 17].

Trispecific CTLs administered prophylactically has demonstrated CMV-specific reactivity in 70% of patients with no increase in the incidence of GVHD. CMV- and EBV-specific T cell numbers rise in the absence of viral reactivation, but adenoviral-CTL expansion is only observed in the context of adenoviral infection. More recent studies have used nucleofection to introduce DNA plasmids encoding multiple immunogenic antigens from CMV, EBV, and adenovirus into APCs, or have used viral antigen–derived 15-mer peptide libraries (pepmix) with APCs to deliver a product with a broader CMV-reactive T cell repertoire [10, 16, 17].

16. Conclusion

Increased numbers of both systemic and upper respiratory tract viral infections occur post-transplant due to ineffective immune reconstitution. Early diagnosis and treatment are critically important to reduce morbidity and mortality associated with these infections. Viral infections cause morbidity and mortality in these immunosuppressed patients due to inability of the host immune system to limit viral replication and dissemination, and loss of T cell function is central to this effect. Immunotherapeutic strategies to accelerate reconstitution of virus-specific immunity and to hasten T cell recovery after transplants remain a compelling alternative to drug treatments. CMV- and EBV-directed virus-specific T cells (VSTs) are being used in the settings of profound immunosuppressed SOT and ASCT patients. Emerging evidence supports the use of VSTs for treatment of broader range of viral targets, including varicella-zoster virus, adenovirus, and BK virus [10, 14–17].

Abbreviation

EBV	Epstein Barr Virus
PTLD	post-transplant Lymphoproliferative disorder
IST	immunosuppression
HHV6	human Herpes simplex virus 6

BK	BK polyoma virus
HSV	Herpes simplex virus
VZV	Varicella Zoster virus
PCR	polymerase chain reaction
CSF	cerebrospinal fluid
IVIG	intravenous immunoglobulin

Author details

Seema Naik*, Kevin Rakszawski, Joseph Cioccio, Hong Zheng and Hiroko Shike
Penn State Cancer Institute, Milton Hershey Medical Center, Hershey, PA, USA

*Address all correspondence to: snaik@pennstatehealth.psu.edu

References

[1] Brunstein CG, Weisdorf DJ, DeFor T, et al. Marked increased risk of Epstein-Barr virus related complications with the addition of antithymocyte globulin to a nonmyeloablative conditioning prior to unrelated umbilical cord blood transplantation. Blood. 2006;**108**: 2874-2880

[2] Xu LP, Zhang CL, Mo XD, et al. Epstein-Barr virus-related post-transplantation lymphoproliferative disorder after unmanipulated human leukocyte antigen haploidentical hematopoietic stem cell transplantation: Incidence, risk factors, treatment, and clinical outcomes. Biology of Blood and Marrow Transplantation. 2015;**21**(12):2185-2191

[3] Barker JN, Doubrovina E, Sauter C, et al. Successful treatment of EBV-associated post transplantation lymphoma after cord blood transplantation using third-party EBV-specific cytotoxic T lymphocytes. Blood. 2 December 2010;**116**(23):5045-5049. DOI: 10.1182/blood-2010-04-281873

[4] Naik S, Riches M, Hari P, et al. Survival outcomes of allogeneic hematopoietic cell transplants with EBV-positive or EBV-negative post-transplant lymphoproliferative disorder, A CIBMTR study. Transplant Infectious Disease. 2019;**21**(5):e1314

[5] Ballen KK, Koreth J, Chen YB, et al. Selection of optimal alternative graft source: Mismatched unrelated donor, umbilical cord blood, or haploidentical transplant. Blood. 2012;**119**(9):1972-1980

[6] van Esser JW, Niesters HG, van der Holt B, et al. Prevention of Epstein-Barr virus-lymphoproliferative disease by molecular monitoring and preemptive rituximab in high-risk patients after allogeneic stem cell transplantation. Blood. 15 June 2002;**99**(12):4364-4369

[7] Worth A, Conyers R, Cohen J, et al. Pre-emptive rituximab based on viremia and T cell reconstitution: A highly effective strategy for the prevention of Epstein–Barr virus-associated lymphoproliferative disease following stem cell transplantation. British Journal of Hematology. 2011;**155**:377-385

[8] Cesaro S, Murrone A, Mengoli C, et.al. The real-time polymerase chain reaction-guided modulation of immunosuppression enables the pre-emptive management of Epstein–Barr virus reactivation after allogeneic hematopoietic stem cell transplantation. British Journal of Haematology. 2005;**128**:224-233

[9] Atilla E, Atilla PA, Bozdağ SC, et al. A review of infectious complications after haploidentical hematopoietic stem cell transplantations. Infection. 2017;**45**(4):403-411

[10] Christin LAM, Myers GD, et al. Cytotoxic T lymphocyte therapy with donor T cells prevents and treats adenovirus and Epstein-Barr virus infections after haploidentical and matched unrelated stem cell transplantation. Blood. 2009;**114**(19):4283-4292

[11] Mulanovich VE, Jiang Y, de Lima M, Shpall EJ, Champlin RE, Ciurea SO. Infectious complications in cord blood and T-cell depleted haploidentical stem cell transplantation. American Journal of Blood Research. 2011;**1**(1):98-105

[12] La Casce AS. Post-transplant lymphoproliferative disorders. The Oncologist. 2006;**11**(6):674-680

[13] Parody R, Martino R, Rovira M, et al. Severe infections after unrelated donor allogeneic hematopoietic stem cell transplantation in adults: Comparison of cord blood

transplantation with peripheral blood and bone marrow transplantation. Biology of Blood and Marrow Transplantation. 2006;**12**(7):734-748

[14] Abbas S, Raybould JE, Sastry S, de la Cruz O. Respiratory viruses in transplant recipients: More than just a cold. Clinical syndromes and infection prevention principles. International Journal of Infectious Diseases. 2017;**62**:86-93

[15] Schmidt ME, Varga SM. The CD8 T cell response to respiratory virus infections. Frontiers in Immunology. 2018;**9**:678. DOI: 10.3389/fimmu.2018.00678

[16] O'Reilly R, Prockop S, Hasan A, et al. Virus-specific T-cell banks for 'off the shelf' adoptive therapy of refractory infections. Bone Marrow Transplantation. 2016;**51**:1163-1172

[17] Roddie C, Peggs KS. Immunotherapy for transplantation-associated viral infections. The Journal of Clinical Investigation. 2017;**127**(7):2513-2522

[18] Lindemans CA, Leen AM, Boelens JJ. How I treat adenovirus in hematopoietic stem cell transplant recipients. Blood. 2010;**116**(25):5476-5485. DOI: 10.1182/blood-2010-04-259291

[19] Dropulic LK, Jones RJ. Polyomavirus BK infection in blood and marrow transplant recipients. Bone Marrow Transplantation. 2008;**41**(1):11-18

[20] Cesaro S, Dalianis T, Rinaldo CH, et al. ECIL guidelines for the prevention, diagnosis and treatment of BK polyomavirus-associated hemorrhagic cystitis in hematopoietic stem cell transplant recipients. Journal of Antimicrobial Chemotherapy. 2018;**73**(1):12-21

[21] Dykewicz CA, Jaffe HW, Kaplan JE, et al. Guidelines for preventing opportunistic infections among hematopoietic stem cell transplant recipients. Recommendations of CDC, the infectious disease society of America, and the American society of blood and marrow transplantation. MMWR. 20 October 2000;**49**(RR10):1-128

[22] Ljungman P et al. Prevention and treatment of viral infections in stem cell transplant recipients. British Journal of Hematology. 2002;**118**:44-57

[23] Boeckh M, Kim HW, Flowers ME, Meyers JD, Bowden RA. Long-term acyclovir for prevention of Varicella zoster virus disease after allogeneic hematopoietic cell transplantation—A randomized double-blind placebo-controlled study. Blood. 2006;**107**(5):1800-1805. DOI: 10.1182/blood-2005-09-3624

Chapter 5

The New Era of Immunotherapy in Bile Duct Cancer Management

Cosmas Rinaldi Adithya Lesmana and Baiq Kirana D. Mandasari

Abstract

Bile duct carcinoma or well known as cholangiocarcinoma (CCA) is the second most common of primary liver malignancy after hepatocellular carcinoma (HCC). Although cholangiocarcinoma is a rare cancer, it has an aggressive feature with very poor prognosis. The epidemiological profile of cholangiocarcinoma varies widely across the world, which is reflecting the exposure of different risk factors, such as chronic inflammatory disease of the biliary tract, specific infectious disease, and congenital malformation. Diagnosis of CCA is quite challenging. CCA is generally asymptomatic in the early stages. Therefore, the management of this malignancy is often delayed due to late diagnosed, where the metastasis has already present or even when it is causing bile duct obstruction. Treatment for CCA is often difficult and should be managed in the tertiary referral hospital with a multidisciplinary team approach. Surgical treatment with complete resection could be benefit only for patient with early stage of the disease. Other treatment modalities as adjuvant therapy are also have been developed to improve survival of the patient, such as chemotherapy, radiotherapy, molecular targeted therapy, targeting angiogenesis and EGFR, and immunotherapy. Recently, immunotherapy has also been developed as a new cancer treatment option and showed a promising result. Whether immunotherapy can be useful for treatment biliary malignancy is still controversial. Hence, a lot of studies is still required to confirm the preliminary findings.

Keywords: bile duct carcinoma, bile duct carcinoma management, immunotherapy, gastroenterology

1. Introduction

The bile duct carcinoma or known as cholangiocarcinoma (CCA) by the definition is a malignancy that originate from cholangiocytes lining the biliary tree. It is included in liver malignancy and become the second most common primary liver malignancy after hepatocellular carcinoma. [1, 2] Incidence of this malignancy is 10–20% cases of all hepatic cancer. [2, 3] Although cholangiocarcinoma is a rare cancer, it has an aggressive feature with very poor prognosis. The data showed that the incidence of cholangiocarcinoma among gastrointestinal cancer approximately reaches 3% but has nearly 20% of death from all hepatobiliary cancer. [3, 4] In addition, cholangiocarcinoma is a clinically silent disease at early stage. Therefore, the diseases are usually diagnosed at advanced stage with poor prognosis.

CCA may occur anywhere in the biliary tract, however, based on where the tumor arises in the biliary tree, it is classified into intrahepatic (iCCA) and extrahepatic bile duct cholangiocarcinoma (eCCA). Extrahepatic bile duct cholangiocarcinoma is divided into two types, perihilar (pCCA) and distal (dCCA) cholangiocarcinoma. iCCAs arises above the second - order of the bile ducts. In contrary, the point anatomical which is distinction pCCA and dCCA is the insertion of the cystic duct. The majority of cholangiocarcinoma are in the perihilar (50–60% cases) and distal region (20–30% cases), and only 10% of CCA are located in intrahepatic. [5]

The tumor is considered rare in most countries with incidence rate from 2001 to 2015 was 1.26 cases per 100,000 persons and has a mortality rate 1–6 per 100,000. [1, 6] Nevertheless, this malignancy is still an endemic disease with high prevalence and incidence in some countries or regions such as Thailand and South Korea. The epidemiological profile of cholangiocarcinoma varies widely across the world, which is reflecting the exposure of different risk factor, such as chronic inflammatory disease of the biliary tract, specific infectious disease, and congenital malformation. In western countries, primary sclerosing cholangitis (PSC) causing biliary obliterative fibrosis, is the major etiology of CCA. [7] Specific in endemic area, Northeast Thailand, with incidence rate 118.5 per 100.000, which is 100 times higher than the global rate. [8] Number of mortality cases from liver and bile duct cancer is the leading cause of death in Thai males and places the third place in female with total number 28.000 deaths per year. [9] Northeast region of Thailand showed the highest number of liver mortality, comprising 70% of cases. [9] In this area, incidence of CCA is strongly related to liver fluke infestation that is endemic in Mekong River. Liver fluke infection is caused by water-borne parasites known as *Opisthorchis viverrini*, *Clonorchis sinensis*, and *Opisthorchis feluneus*. These parasites are transmitted to human by the consumption of raw, pickled, or undercooked infected fish associated with local tradition and poor income. [10–12]

The life cycle of this parasite is quite complex, involving two intermediate host (snail to fish) and including several changes of morphological feature. Fish contaminated with metacercaria is ingested by the human. [2] Infected human excretes the egg produced by the mature adult worms in their feces. [2, 13] Feces then contaminated the fresh water and then ingested by snail and the larva develop and hatch in the digestive tract of the snail. [2, 13] After that, thousands of cercariae were excreted into the water and penetrate the skin fish, encyst, and forming metacercaria. In the body of human, this parasite excyst in the duodenum and ascend to the bile duct via the ampulla of Vater then migrate further into the smaller and proximal bile duct, then become mature worm and able to sexually produce. [2, 13] Adult worm could survive up to 25 years in the biliary tree and causing mild symptoms such as malaise, abdominal discomfort, and diarrhea. Long term complication of this infection associated with hepatomegaly, chronic infection, cholecystitis, gallstone, and periportal fibrosis. [2, 13] Long term of chronic inflammation found to be a major etiological precursor of hepatobiliary malignancy, predominantly of CCA. Once a person is infected and suffered from chronic infection and inflammation, the risk for having CCA is increasing and could present within 30–40 years after infection. [11] Until now, the prognosis of CCA is remain poor and death tend to occur within 3–6 months after diagnosis. [11] There are several hypothesizes on the mechanism or pathway how the chronic infection could develop become malignancy: 1) mechanical damage caused by the fluke sucker, 2) fluke toxic secretary product, and 3) immunopathological host response. [11] These pathways then caused proliferative response and formation of precursor lesion such as epithelial and adenomatous hyperplasia, and goblet cell metaplasia. [11]

Beside parasite infection, primary sclerosing cholangitis (PSC) is another common etiology of cholangiocarcinoma, especially in the western population. PSC is a progressive cholestatic biliary characterized by the chronic inflammation that leads to destruction of the intra and extrahepatic bile duct. [14] The incidence rate of PSC ranges from 0 to 1.3 per 100.000 people. [15] At early stage, PSC is asymptomatic and is usually already diagnosed at advanced stage whereas jaundice and pruritus are the major complaint due to cholestasis. It has been also strongly associated with inflammatory bowel disease (IBD). On the other hand, PSC is often found with portal hypertension, cirrhosis, and in hepatobiliary and colorectal malignancies. [16, 17]

The other risk factor for developing CCA is biliary stones which is formed in the biliary tree, substantially in intrahepatic bile duct or known as hepatolithiasis. Biliary stones are typically concomitant with biliary stasis, cholangitis, strictures, and bacterial infection, leading to long term inflammation and biliary injury, and at the end, increasing the risk of malignant cholangiocytes growth. [18] Abnormal morphological also increase the risk for malignant transformation. Choledochal cysts is a rare congenital malformation characterized by dilatation of the biliary tree, can be single or multiple, and can be developed in the intra or extra hepatic bile ducts. [17, 19] Moreover, the coincidence of abnormal pancreatobiliary duct junctions increases the possibility of cholangiocarcinogenesis. This due to pancreatic enzyme reflux, cholestasis, and elevated bile acid concentrations. [19]

Exposure to chemical carcinogens such as Thorotrast, halogenated hydrocarbon solvent, and 1,2-dichloropropane were found to be associated with CCA incidence. [20, 21] Carcinogens-induced liver insult has been showed to promote hepatocyte remodeling, genomic instability, DNA methylation, and disrupt the liver architecture. Moreover, some studies reported few genetic mutations related to hepatobiliary malignancy. [22] Hepatic disease associated with CCA include alcoholic liver disease, cirrhosis, and cholangitis are included become risk factor. [17]

Diagnosis of CCA is quite challenging. CCA is generally asymptomatic in the early stage. Therefore, management of this malignancy is often delayed due to late diagnosed, where it already metastasis or compress the bile duct. The clinical features of CCA are heterogenous, with general malaise, cachexia, abdominal pain, night sweats, fatigue, weight loss, asthenia, and/or jaundice which is more frequent symptom in pCCA and dCCA due to biliary tract obstruction. [23, 24] Diagnosis of CCA is usually confirmed by combining nonspecific biomarkers in serum, biopsy specimens, and imaging technique. To date, there is no specific serum marker available for diagnosing CCA. Liver function parameters such as serum bilirubin, alkaline phosphatase, and aminotransferase enzyme usually elevate when biliary obstruction is presence. [24, 25] However, it is not specific signs for biliary malignancy. Serum tumor marker such as carbohydrate antigen (CA) 19–9, CA-125, and carcinoembryonic antigen (CEA) are the most widely used markers for suspected CCA. [25] But this diagnostic tool should not be used alone due to their poor diagnostic performance and inherent limitations.

Imaging techniques which are required to help diagnosis CCA are trans-abdominal ultrasonography (US), contrast-enhanced ultrasonography (CEUS), CT scan, and MRI. Becoming diagnostic tools, imaging techniques play a key role in the management of CCA in term of diagnosis, staging, follow-up, and assessment of favorable treatment response. The accuracy of diagnosis is depending on the anatomical location and growth pattern of CCA. Magnetic resonance cholangiopancreatography (MRCP) has the higher diagnostic accuracy for sizing strictures and localizing. [24, 25]

But unfortunately, there are no specific CCA radiology pattern exists. Therefore, histopathology or cytological analysis is also necessary for confirming the diagnosis. Definitive diagnosis is usually made by undergoing endoscopic retrograde cholangiopancreatography (ERCP) procedure for fluid cytology, brush cytology, fluorescence in situ hybridization (FISH), and cholangioscope or chromoendoscopy-guided biopsy. [26–28] Those multiple diagnostic modalities are required to 1) establish strictures anatomical location; 2) distinguish between benign and malignant strictures; 3) differentiate CCA from gallbladder cancer; 4) stage and grade the tumor; and 5) plan treatment approach. Based on WHO classification of biliary tract cancer it is showing an adenocarcinoma or mucinous carcinoma, with tubular and/or papillary structures and a variable fibrous stroma. [24, 25]

Determine staging of CCA is important for choosing the treatment, its resectability, and the outcome of the treatment. TNM classification system of American Joint Committee on Cancer (AJCC) and Union for International Cancer Control (UICC) has been used at present to determine the staging of CCA. TNM staging system is based on imaging tests which is evaluating the number of primary nodules, vascular invasion, direct extension in neighboring tissue, and bile duct involvement. [29] pCCA can be further divided according to the Bismuth-Corlette classification, depending on the size of the tumor, disease extension in the main bile duct, hepatic artery and/or portal involvement, lymph node involvement, distant metastasis, and remnant liver volume after resection. [30] iCCA could be classified based on 3 growth pattern which has different prognosis of each pattern: mass-forming (MF-iCCA), periductal infiltration (PI-iCCA), and intraductal growth (IG-iCCA). [31]

Treatment for managing cholangiocarcinoma is quite difficult too and should be managed in the tertiary hospital with a multidisciplinary team experienced in endoscopic, percutaneous, and surgical approaches. Management of this malignancy also depends on the staging of the tumor. Surgical treatment with complete resection could give benefit only for patient with early stage of the disease [32].

Resection could be performed in approximately 30% of patient with CCA. This is the only option that provides a real possibility for long-term survival in patient diagnosed with CCA. The indication and extension of surgery are determined based on clinical features of the patient, functional liver reserve, and the location and extension of the tumor, which include the association with vascular structure and negative metastatic disease. [33, 34]

Criteria for patients who are considered as absolute unresectability are the presence of nonresectable extrahepatic, hepatic metastases, bilateral extension of the tumor with involvement of the secondary biliary tract, complete occlusion of the main portal vein, thrombosis in portal vein contralateral to the tumor. [23] The most common postoperative complications are hemorrhage, infection, liver failure, cardiorespiratory failure, and adrenal failure. Mortality and morbidity for postoperative patient are still remaining high, 8,2% and 50%, respectively. [35] In several condition, drainage should be applied. But in the recent years, increasing number of patients with unresectable intrahepatic and extrahepatic CCA are being included to be candidate for liver transplant. Other treatment modalities as adjuvant therapy are also developed to improve the survival of the patient, such as chemotherapy, radiotherapy, molecular targeted therapy, targeting angiogenesis and EGFR, and immunotherapy.

2. Role of immunotherapy in cancer management

2.1 History and definition

Cancer immunotherapy is significantly progressing and rapidly advancing. In the recent years, immunotherapy is considered to be the fifth pillar of cancer therapy and management modality besides surgery, cytotoxic chemotherapy, radiation, and targeted therapy. The mechanism of immunotherapy in cancer management is to determine a manipulation of the immune system by using immune agents such as vaccine, cytokine, cell therapies and humoral, transfection agent. Cancer immunotherapy has to stimulate the host anti-tumor response by increasing the effector cell number and production of soluble mediators, decrease the host's suppressor mechanism by inducing tumor killing environment, and could modulate immune checkpoint. [36, 37]

In 1891, William Coley, who is known today as the Father of Immunotherapy, injected heat inactivated bacteria or known as Coley toxins to the sarcoma patient who was inoperable. [38] This first experiment resulted in long term regression of the sarcoma after an erysipelas infection after injecting the toxin. [38] By late 1970s, immunotherapy for managing cancer was discovered. The first experiment was done in bladder cancer case which is managed by using BCG (Bacillus Calmette-Guerin). Then, it is continued with IFN therapy in malignant melanoma. [39] Brief background review of immune system is classically considered to be comprised of the innate and adaptive arms. Immune system which are included in innate immune system are dendritic cells, natural killer cells (NK), macrophages, neutrophils, eosinophils, basophils, and mast cells. As we known, this group of immune system does not need prior stimulation by antigen, and it plays role as first line of defense against foreign antigens. In the contrary, adaptive immune system consists of B lymphocytes, CD4 helper T lymphocytes, and CD 8 cytotoxic T lymphocytes (CTLs). This group of immune system requires formal presentation by antigen presenting cells (APCs) for its activation. [40, 41]

Several kinds of malignant cells are able to evade the tumor immunosurveillance system by manipulating their own characteristic as well as the cells in their microenvironment to become successful tumors. The concept that the immune system is capable for detecting and killing nascent non-self-malignant cells was developed. Elimination, equilibrium, and escape are three main phases of immunoediting process. [42] The elimination phase is the initial damage process and destruction of the tumor cell by innate immune system, then tumor antigens are presented to the dendritic cells, followed by presentation to the T cell and then create tumor-specific CD4 and CD8 T-cells. Second phase occurs when tumor cells survive after the initial destruction but are not able to progress and being maintained in an equilibrium state. The last phase is escape phase. [42] In this phase, tumor cells are growing rapidly, followed by metastasize of tumor cell due to loss control of the immune system and the tumor cells do not presented antigens on its surface or even losing their MHC class1 expression. Tumor cell could protect their self from T cell by expressing immune checkpoint (IC) molecules on their surface. [42]

The ability of this malignant cells to evade immune destruction by modulating its own cellular characteristic and creating its own "tumor microenvironment" by recruiting apparently normal immune cells to help shield it from attack of immune system. In addition, tumor cell can influence the systemic environment by altering hematopoiesis and tissue parenchyma of organs at distant sites. Cancer immunotherapies play role in manipulating these tumor microenvironments. But the loss of MHC class 1 expression manipulating is remaining challenge. [43–45]

First, older, and non-specific immunotherapies are the kind of immune stimulator cytokines such as interleukin-2 IL-2) and interferon (IFN). [46] Beside that, synthetic analogue of bacterial cell wall called L-MTP could activate monocytes and macrophages is one of the immunostimulatory cytokines. Vaccine trials using multiple neoantigens specific to and individual patient's tumor have shown promising results in two small early trials with the aim to expose patients to those tumor antigens which can provoke an antitumor immune response via the generation of tumor specific antibodies and T cells. [46] BCG was the first vaccine used as cancer immunotherapy for treating bladder carcinoma. [47]

Oncolytic viruses are the combination of biologic therapy and immunotherapy. Viruses which are used for this method has genetically modified to lack virulence against normal cell but has a selective feature to invade and lyse cancer cells. Viral-induced tumor cell destruction undergoing further attack by an immune system. [48]

Adoptive cell therapy (ACT) is one type of immunotherapy which involves in the isolation and in-vitro expansion of tumor-specific T-cells, which is given through infusion in the cancer patient. ACT using NK cells could be used to treat solid tumor metastasis and hematological cancers. [49] Several forms of ACT using different techniques are culturing tumor infiltrating lymphocytes directly from the tumor, isolating and expanding one particular T-cell or the clone, using T cell which have been engineered in vitro so that it could recognize and attack the tumor cells or known as chimeric antigen receptor T-cell (CAR T-cell) therapy. ACT has produced remarkable result in clinical trials with melanoma and hematologic malignancies. But some studies reported death have occurred in the trial phase due to cytokine release syndrome or cytokine storm. [50]

Another immunotherapy, Immune checkpoint, work by targeting molecules that serve as checks in the regulation of immune responses and block inhibitory molecules or activate stimulatory molecules and enhance pre-existing anti-cancer immune response. [51]

2.2 The clinical importance of immunotherapy

Cancer immunotherapy works to stimulate the host's anti-tumor response. The mechanism included are increasing the effector cell number and production of soluble mediators, decreasing the host's suppressor mechanism by inducing tumor killing environment, and modulating immune checkpoints. The usefulness of cancer immunotherapy was introduced in the beginning to manage bladder cancer. The overall 5-year survival after transmitting immunotherapy is 77%. [39] Patients with moderate and high-grade bladder cancer who received intravesical immunotherapy with BCG have shown good result. Immune checkpoint inhibitors showed a promising clinical research in managing anti-cancer immune responses. Several studies using Nivolumab, Ipilimumab, and Pertuzumab are still on progress in metastatic bladder cancer. Some cytokines which are messenger molecules, play a role to control the growth and activity of immune system cells. [52] Treatment using cytokines as immunotherapy can enhance the activity of the immune system against tumors. The link of IL-2 to the antibody, ALT-801, and cytokines can target IL-2 to cancer cells. [53] Oncolytic virus therapy could also be used to treat bladder cancer using adenovirus which expresses the immune stimulating cytokine GM-CSF. [54]

Immunotherapy is developed to manage some immunogenic cancer cases besides bladder cancer. The using of immunotherapy for managing breast cancer have been improved and approved in the recent years. Although the best treatment of breast cancer is surgery, but combination therapy followed by chemotherapy, radiation therapy, or immunotherapy could increase clinical outcome for patient. A promising immunotherapy using immune checkpoint inhibitors that work by targeting molecules that serve as checks in the regulation of immune response and block inhibitory molecules or activate stimulatory molecules. [39] The other form of immunotherapy which can be used for breast cancer is monoclonal antibodies and adoptive T cell transfer. By definition, adoptive T cell transfer is a process of removing T cell from the patient, then it would be modified genetically or treated with chemical to enhance its activity and re-introduced into the patient. Specifically, in breast cancer, T cell genetically is modified to target the carcinoembryonic antigen (CEA). [55]

Another immunogenic cancer is cervical cancer caused by infection of human papillomavirus (HPV). Cervical cancer is the third most frequent cancer among women in the world. [56] The prevalence of this cancer is decreasing due to development widespread of screening tools Pap test and vaccine to prevent HPV infection. In the recent years, monoclonal antibodies, checkpoint inhibitor, and adoptive T cell transfer have become additional therapy for managing progressivity of cancer cell. [39]

Immunotherapies are also developed as a new modality treatment to treat brain cancer, colorectal cancer, esophageal cancer, and biliary tract cancer. Probably, in time, immunotherapy could lead to personalized medicine that will increase overall survival and progression free survival for many treatments. [39]

2.3 The role of immunotherapy in managing bile duct malignancy

Biliary tract malignancy is an invasive carcinoma which can be originated from gallbladder or bile duct. It has been known that the immune system in human body has a significant role in the surveillance and eradication of cancer cells. Tumor that lack the mismatch repair system harbor more mutation than tumor without this deficiency. Thus, the neoantigen generated and be recognize as immunogenic antigen. The characteristic of mismatch repair deficient tumors is microsatellite instability (MSI). There are approximately 3% of CCA are mismatch repair-deficient/MSI-high. [56] This feature makes the tumor cells are susceptible to programmed cell death protein 1 (PD-1) inhibitors. Zhu et al. studied about efficacy and safety of gemcitabine, oxaliplatin, and bevacizumab in advanced biliary-tract cancers and the correlation of changes in 18-fluorodeoxyglucose PET with clinical outcome in a phase 2 study showed that combination of chemotherapy and immunotherapy have anti-tumor effect with tolerable safety and promising efficacy for managing advanced biliary tract malignancy. This combination treatment was generally well tolerated with less adverse event and manageable toxicity. [57]

Another clinical data about immune-directed therapy in CCA is still scanty. Vaccine for preventing CCA has been developed and tested but no data has showed successful result. [58] CAR T cell immunotherapy in recent years has been developed. Guo et al. in their study about expanded and parallel clinical trial of EGFR-specific chimeric antigen receptor-engineered autologous T (CART) cell immunotherapy. The aim of this study is to assess the safety and activity of CART-EGFR cell therapy in EGFR-positive advanced unresectable, relapsed/metastatic biliary tract cancer. Total sample of this study is 19 patients and showed that CART-EGFR cell infusion was tolerated, 1 achieved complete response and 10 achieved stable disease. We can conclude that CART-EGFR cell immunotherapy was a safe and active strategy for EGFR-positive advanced biliary tract cancer. [59] Wei et al. showed that in some patients, immune checkpoint blockade using monoclonal antibodies has shown remarkable and durable response rate in a many kind of malignancy cell. [60] Le et al. in their study concluded that mismatch-repair status predicted clinical benefit of immune checkpoint blockade with pembrolizumab and achieving objective responses in up to 40% of patients. [61] Study by Ott et al. in KEYNOTE-028 basket trial of pembrolizumab included patients with advanced biliary tract cancer resulted the objective response rate was 17% with median progression-free survival of 1.8 months. [62] However, further studies are required either combination immunotherapeutic approaches targeting both the innate and adaptive immune system or combined strategies involving chemotherapy or radiation.

3. Conclusions

Bile duct cancer is still one of the challenging malignancies in the gastroenterology field due to the difficulty in early detection and most of patients come in the late stage of the disease. Chemotherapy is still the main option of management despite surgery and biliary drainage. Immunotherapy is a promising treatment option in the future; however, further studies would be needed to give strong evidence before it can be used in common clinical practice.

Author details

Cosmas Rinaldi Adithya Lesmana[1,2*] and Baiq Kirana D. Mandasari[1]

1 Division of Hepatobiliary, Department of Internal Medicine, Dr. Cipto Mangunkusumo National General Hospital, Medical Faculty Universitas Indonesia, Jakarta, Indonesia

2 Digestive Disease and GI Oncology Centre, Medistra Hospital, Jakarta, Indonesia

*Address all correspondence to: medicaldr2001id@yahoo.com

References

[1] Patel N, Benipal B. Incidence of cholangiocarcinoma in the USA from 2001 to 2015: a US cancer statistics analysis of 50 states. Cureus. 2019;11(1):e3962. Published 2019 Jan 25. doi:10.7759/cureus.3962

[2] Alsaleh M, Leftley Z, Barbera TA, et al. Cholangiocarcinoma: a guide for the nonspecialist. Int J Gen Med. 2018;12:13-23. Published 2018 Dec 20. doi:10.2147/IJGM.S186854

[3] Shaib Y, El-Serag HB. The epidemiology of cholangiocarcinoma. Semin Liver Dis. 2004;24(2):115-125

[4] Kirstein MM, Vogel A: Epidemiology and risk factors of cholangiocarcinoma. Visc Med. 2016, 32:395-400. 10.1159/000453013

[5] Banales JM, Marin JJG, Lamarca A, et al. Cholangiocarcinoma 2020: the next horizon in mechanisms and management [published online ahead of print, 2020 Jun 30]. Nat Rev Gastroenterol Hepatol. 2020;10.1038/s41575-020-0310-z. doi:10.1038/s41575-020-0310-z

[6] Global Burden of Disease Cancer Collaboration; Fitzmaurice C, Dicker D, et al. The global Burden of cancer 2013. JAMA Oncol 2015; 1: 505-527 [PMID: 26181261 DOI: 10.1001/jamaoncol.2015.0735]

[7] Massarweh NN, El-Serag HB. Epidemiology of Hepatocellular Carcinoma and Intrahepatic Cholangiocarcinoma. Cancer Control 2017; 24: 1073274817729245 [PMID: 28975830 DOI: 10.1177/1073274817729245]

[8] Bragazzi M, Cardinale V, Carpino G. Cholangiocarcinoma: epidemiology and risk factors. Transl Gastrointest Cancer. 2012;1(1):21-32.

[9] Sripa B, Pairojkul C. Cholangiocarcinoma: lessons from Thailand. Curr Opin Gastroenterol. 2008;24(3):349-356

[10] Ziegler AD, Petney TN, Grundy-Warr C, et al. Dams and disease triggers on the lower Mekong river. PLoS Negl Trop Dis. 2013;7(6): e2166

[11] Sripa B, Kaewkes S, Sithithaworn P, et al. Liver fluke induces cholangiocarcinoma. PLoS Med. 2007;4(7):e201.

[12] Sithithaworn P, Andrews RH, Nguyen VD, et al. The current status of opisthorchiasis and clonorchiasis in the Mekong Basin. Parasitol Int. 2012;61(1):10-16.

[13] Kaewpitoon N, Kaewpitoon SJ, Pengsaa P, Sripa B. Opisthorchis viverrini: the carcinogenic human liver fluke. World J Gastroenterol. 2008;14(5):666-674.

[14] Karlsen TH, Boberg KM. Update on primary sclerosing cholangitis. J Hepatol. 2013;59(3):571-582.

[15] Boonstra K, Beuers U, Ponsioen CY. Epidemiology of primary sclerosing cholangitis and primary biliary cirrhosis: a systematic review. J Hepatol. 2012;56(5):1181-1188

[16] Lindor KD, Kowdley KV, Harrison ME, American College of Gastroenterology. ACG clinical guideline: primary sclerosing cholangitis. Am J Gastroenterol. 2015;110(5):646-659.

[17] Tyson GL, El-Serag HB. Risk factors for cholangiocarcinoma. Hepatology. 2011;54(1):173-184.

[18] Kim HJ, Kim JS, Joo MK, et al. Hepatolithiasis and intrahepatic cholangiocarcinoma: a review.

World J Gastroenterol. 2015;21(48): 13418-13431.

[19] Söreide K, Körner H, Havnen J, Söreide JA. Bile duct cysts in adults. Br J Surg. 2004;91(12):1538-1548

[20] Kato I, Kido C. Increased risk of death in Thorotrast-exposed patients during the late follow-up period. Jpn J Cancer Res. 1987;78(11): 1187-1192.

[21] Kumagai S, Kurumatani N, Arimoto A, Ichihara G. Cholangiocarcinoma among offset colour proof-printing workers exposed to 1,2-dichloropropane and/or dichloromethane. Occup Environ Med. 2013;70(7):508-510

[22] Wang L, Liu D, Shimizu T, Fukumoto M. Mechanisms of liver carcinogenesis by chronic exposure to alpha-particles form internally deposited Thorotrast. Int Congr Ser. 2005;1276:192-194

[23] Huguet JM, Lobo M, Labrador JM, et al. Diagnostic-therapeutic management of bile duct cancer. World J Clin Cases. 2019;7(14):1732-1752. doi:10.12998/wjcc.v7.i14.1732

[24] Khan SA, Davidson BR, Goldin RD, et al. Guidelines for the diagnosis and treatment of cholangiocarcinoma: an update. Gut. 2012;61(12):1657-1669

[25] van Beers BE. Diagnosis of cholangiocarcinoma. HPB (Oxford). 2008;10(2):87-93

[26] Romagnuolo J, Bardou M, Rahme E, Joseph L, Reinhold C, Barkun AN. Magnetic resonance cholangiopancreatography: a meta-analysis of test performance in suspected biliary disease. Ann Intern Med 2003; 139: 547-557 [PMID: 14530225]

[27] Chapman R, Fevery J, Kalloo A, Nagorney DM, Boberg KM, Shneider B, Gores GJ; American Association for the Study of Liver Diseases. Diagnosis and management of primary sclerosing cholangitis. Hepatology 2010; 51: 660-678 [PMID: 20101749 DOI: 10.1002/hep.23294]

[28] Mansour JC, Aloia TA, Crane CH, Heimbach JK, Nagino M, Vauthey JN. Hilar cholangiocarcinoma: expert consensus statement. HPB (Oxford) 2015; 17: 691-699 [PMID: 26172136 DOI: 10.1111/hpb.12450]

[29] Amin MB, Greene FL, Edge SB, Compton CC, Gershenwald JE, Brookland RK, Meyer L, Gress DM, Byrd DR, Winchester DP. The Eighth Edition AJCC Cancer Staging Manual: Continuing to build a bridge from a population-based to a more "personalized" approach to cancer staging. CA Cancer J Clin 2017; 67: 93-99 [PMID: 28094848 DOI: 10.3322/caac.21388]

[30] Bismuth H, Corlette MB. Intrahepatic cholangioenteric anastomosis in carcinoma of the hilus of the liver. Surg Gynecol Obstet 1975; 140: 170-178 [PMID: 1079096]

[31] Banales JM, Cardinale V, Carpino G, Marzioni M, Andersen JB, Invernizzi P, Lind GE, Folseraas T, Forbes SJ, Fouassier L, Geier A, Calvisi DF, Mertens JC, Trauner M, Benedetti A, Maroni L, Vaquero J, Macias RI, Raggi C, Perugorria MJ, Gaudio E, Boberg KM, Marin JJ, Alvaro D. Expert consensus document: Cholangiocarcinoma: current knowledge and future perspectives consensus statement from the European Network for the Study of Cholangiocarcinoma (ENS-CCA). Nat Rev Gastroenterol Hepatol 2016; 13: 261-280 [PMID: 27095655 DOI: 10.1038/nrgastro.2016.51]

[32] He P, Shi JS, Chen WK, Wang ZR, Ren H, Li H. Multivariate statistical analysis of clinicopathologic factors influencing survival of patients

with bile duct carcinoma. World J Gastroenterol 2002; 8: 943-946 [PMID: 12378647]

[33] Lladó L, Ramos E, Torras J, Fabregat J, Jorba R, Valls C, Julià D, Serrano T, Figueras J, Rafecas A. [Radical resection of a hilar cholangiocarcinoma. Indications and results]. Cir Esp 2008; 83: 139-144 [PMID: 18341903]

[34] He P, Shi JS, Chen WK, Wang ZR, Ren H, Li H. Multivariate statistical analysis of clinicopathologic factors influencing survival of patients with bile duct carcinoma. World J Gastroenterol 2002; 8: 943-946 [PMID: 12378647]

[35] Esnaola NF, Meyer JE, Karachristos A, Maranki JL, Camp ER, Denlinger CS. Evaluation and management of intrahepatic and extrahepatic cholangiocarcinoma. Cancer 2016; 122: 1349-1369 [PMID: 26799932 DOI: 10.1002/cncr.29692]

[36] Oiseth SJ, Aziz MS. Cancer immunotherapy: a brief review of the history, possibilities, and challenges ahead. J Cancer Metastasis Treat 2017;3:250-261. http://dx.doi.org/10.20517/2394-4722.2017.41

[37] Farkona S, Diamandis EP, Blasutig IM. Cancer immunotherapy: the beginning of the end of cancer?. BMC Med. 2016;14:73. Published 2016 May 5. doi:10.1186/s12916-016-0623-5

[38] Dobosz P, Dzieciątkowski T. The Intriguing History of Cancer Immunotherapy. Front Immunol. 2019;10:2965. Published 2019 Dec 17. doi:10.3389/fimmu.2019.02965

[39] StanculeanuDL,DanielaZ,LazescuA, Bunghez R, Anghel R. Development of new immunotherapy treatments in different cancer types. J Med Life. 2016;9(3):240-248.

[40] Abbas AK, Lichtman AH, Pillai S. Properties and Overview of Immune Responses. In: Cellular and Molecular Immunology, 9th edition. Amsterdam: Elsevier; 2017. p. 1-11.

[41] Brodin P, Davis MM. Human immune system variation. Nat Rev Immunol 2017;17:21-9.

[42] Tsukahara T, Kawaguchi S, Torigoe T, Asanuma H, Nakazawa E, Shimozawa K, Nabeta Y, Kimura S, Kaya M, Nagoya S, Wada T, Yamashita T, Sato N. Prognostic significance of HLA class I expression in osteosarcoma defined by anti-pan HLA class I monoclonal antibody, EMR8-5. Cancer Sc 2006;97:1374-80.

[43] Kitamura T, Qian BZ, Pollard JW. Immune cell promotion of metastasis. Nat Rev Immunol 2015;15:73-86.

[44] McAllister SS, Weinberg RA. The tumour-induced systemic environment as a critical regulator of cancer progression and metastasis. Nat Cell Biol 2014;16:717-27

[45] 40. Garrido F, Aptsiauri N, Doorduijn EM, Garcia Lora AM, van Hall T. The urgent need to recover MHC class I in cancers for effective immunotherapy. Curr Opin Immunol 2016;39:44-51

[46] Kager L, Pötschger U, Bielack S. Review of mifamurtide in the treatment of patients with osteosarcoma. Ther Clin Risk Manag 2010;6:279-86.

[47] Speil C, Rzepka R. Vaccines and vaccine adjuvants as biological response modifiers. Infect Dis Clin North Am 2011;25:755-72.

[48] Choi AH, O'Leary MP, Fong Y, Chen NG. From benchtop to bedside: a review of oncolytic virotherapy. Biomedicines 2016;4:E18.

[49] Guillerey C, Huntington ND, Smyth MJ. Targeting natural killer cells

in cancer immunotherapy. Nat Immunol 2016;17:1025-36.

[50] Jinek M, Chylinski K, Fonfara I, Hauer M, Doudna JA, Charpentier E. A programmable dual-RNA-guided DNA endonuclease in adaptive bacterial immunity. Science 2012;337:816-21.

[51] Sharma P, Hu-Lieskovan S, Wargo JA, Ribas A. Primary, adaptive, and acquired resistance to cancer immunotherapy. Cell 2017;168:70723.

[52] https://clinicaltrials.gov/show/NCT0192 8394 A Phase 1/ 2, Open-label Study of Nivolumab Monotherapy or Nivolumab Combined With Ipilimumab in Subjects With Advanced or Metastatic Solid Tumors, Bristol-Myers Squibb.

[53] Muthuswamy R, Wang L, Pitteroff J, Gingrich JR, Kalinski P. Combination of IFNα and poly-I:C reprograms bladder cancer microenvironment for enhanced CTL attraction. Journal for ImmunoTherapy of Cancer. 2015; 3:6. doi 10.1186/s40425-015-0050-8

[54] Vasekar M, Degraff D, Joshi M. Immunotherapy in Bladder Cancer. Current Molecular Pharmacology. 2015; PMID:26177642

[55] Sabel MS, Arora A, Su G, Chang AE. Adoptive immunotherapy of breast cancer with lymph node cells primed by cryoablation of the primary tumor. December 2006; 53(3):360-366

[56] Le DT, Durham JN, Smith KN, et al. Mismatch repair deficiency predicts response of solid tumors to PD-1 blockade. Science. 2017;357(6349):409-413. doi:10.1126/science.aan6733

[57] Zhu AX, Meyerhardt JA, Blaszkowsky LS, et al. Efficacy and safety of gemcitabine, oxaliplatin, and bevacizumab in advanced biliary-tract cancers and correlation of changes in 18-fluorodeoxyglucose PET with clinical outcome: a phase 2 study. Lancet Oncol. 2010;11(1):48-54. doi:10.1016/S1470-2045(09)70333-X

[58] Yamamoto K, Ueno T, Kawaoka T, et al. MUC1 peptide vaccination in patients with advanced pancreas or biliary tract cancer. Anticancer Res. 2005;25(5):3575-3579

[59] Guo Y, Feng K, Liu Y, et al. Phase I Study of Chimeric Antigen Receptor-Modified T Cells in Patients with EGFR-Positive Advanced Biliary Tract Cancers. Clin Cancer Res. 2018;24(6):1277-1286. doi:10.1158/1078-0432.CCR-17-0432

[60] Wei SC, Duffy CR, Allison JP. Fundamental Mechanisms of Immune Checkpoint Blockade Therapy. Cancer Discov. 2018;8(9):1069-1086. doi:10.1158/2159-8290.CD-18-0367

[61] Le DT, Uram JN, Wang H, et al. PD-1 Blockade in Tumors with Mismatch-Repair Deficiency. N Engl J Med. 2015;372(26):2509-2520. doi:10.1056/NEJMoa1500596

[62] Ott PA, Bang YJ, Piha-Paul SA, et al. T-Cell-Inflamed Gene-Expression Profile, Programmed Death Ligand 1 Expression, and Tumor Mutational Burden Predict Efficacy in Patients Treated With Pembrolizumab Across 20 Cancers: KEYNOTE-028. J Clin Oncol. 2019;37(4):318-327. doi:10.1200/JCO.2018.78.2276

Chapter 6

Role of Hybrid Operating Room: Present and Future

Evan Qize Yuan and Calvin Sze Hang Ng

Abstract

With the dramatic progress of medical imaging modalities and growing needs for high-resolution intraoperative imaging in minimally invasive surgery, hybrid operative room (OR) has been developed as a powerful tool for different surgical scenarios. Under the guidance of high-definition cone beam CT (CBCT), an electromagnetic navigation bronchoscopy (ENB)-based marker implantation and subsequent localization of the pulmonary nodules can be implemented within a hybrid OR. Furthermore, the unparalleled real-time imaging capabilities and the ability to perform multiple tasks within the hybrid OR can facilitate image-guided single-port video-assisted thoracic surgery (iSPVATS), increasing the precision and improving outcomes of the procedure. With the help of a hybrid theatre, catheter-based thermal ablation can provide a safer and less invasive treatment option for select patient groups with early-stage non-small cell lung carcinomas (NSCLC) or metastases. In the future, the combination of hybrid operating room and other inspiring innovative techniques, such as robotic bronchoscopy, 3D-printing, natural orifice transluminal endoscopic surgery (NOTES) lung surgery could lead to a paradigm shift in the way thoracic surgery is conducted.

Keywords: 3-D printing, ablation, cone beam CT, electromagnetic navigation bronchoscopy, hookwire, hybrid operating room, localization, lung cancer, metastases, non-small cell lung carcinoma, natural orifice transluminal endoscopic surgery, robotic bronchoscopy, single-port video-assisted thoracic surgery

1. Introduction

In recent decades, thoracic surgery has undergone revolutionary progress. With the help of imaging technology, surgeons can perform minimally invasive surgery through several small incisions instead of thoracotomy [1]. With the advantages of less pain, quicker recovery, fewer postoperative complications and better cosmesis, minimally invasive surgery has gradually become the mainstream of thoracic disease treatment [2]. Among the many techniques, the single-port video-assisted thoracic surgery (VATS) is becoming more and more popular in recent years [3–5]. When combined with medical imaging techniques and adjuvant instruments, such as computed tomography (CT) guided placement of hookwire/microcoil or dye labeling for localization, the single-port VATS can safely be used to resect lung lesions in a less invasive way [3, 6]. However, there exist some deficiencies in the traditional mode of treatment paradigms, in which the imaging and surgery are operated in separate chambers. The time interval between adjunctive localization techniques conducted under computed tomography guidance and surgery may increase the risk of pneumothorax and wire migration or dislodgement [7]. Moreover, by performing procedures in multiple localities with the risks as described could increase the complexity of care and cost. The emergence of hybrid operating room (OR) provides patients with a less invasive diagnostic and therapeutic option [8]. By conducting the localization and the lung surgery in a hybrid operating room, the rate of pneumothorax, marker dislodgement, and dye diffusion can be minimized, with decreased procedural time and lower costs [3]. More importantly, thoracic surgeons will be able to conduct precise excisions in a much more secure way, even for multifocal lesions, preserving pulmonary tissue and function because of this innovative approach for diagnosing and localizing the nodules [8].

2. What is a hybrid operating room?

The "hybrid operating room (OR)" concept consists of a surgical workspace that integrates imaging devices with a multifunctional surgical table. It allows surgeons to perform diagnostic and therapeutic procedure in a single room, reducing risks caused by delay and patient transfer [9]. Moreover, it is a potentially safer and time-saving option for patients facing different medical situations [10]. Despite its wide utilization in many medical fields, cardiology and vascular surgery in particular, the first hybrid operating room (advanced multimodal image-guided operating [AMIGO] suite) for general thoracic surgery was only reported in 2013 by Professor Raphael Bueno's group at Harvard University, Brigham and Women's Hospital, Boston [11]. Equipped with three functional compartments that incorporate magnetic resonance imaging (MRI), near-infrared imaging, cone-beam computed tomography (CBCT), and positron emission tomography (PET), the 5700-square-feet AMIGO suite is capable of providing sterling real-time imaging of the patients undergoing different types of surgeries.

In the subsequent year, a reduced scale hybrid theater (Artis zeego, Siemens Healthcare GmbH, Erlangen, Germany) was set up in the authors' hospital [12]. Similarly, this suite can provide imaging support for different types of surgical scenarios, making it possible for the surgeons to conduct image-guided electromagnetic navigation bronchoscopy (ENB) and VATS procedures. The robotic C-arm CBCT can move flexibly without affecting the surgical procedure. It is worth mentioning that this operating room has a relatively smaller area (approximately 760 square feet), which is meaningful when it comes to space-saving considerations. The complete content of the hybrid operating room is listed in **Table 1** [12].

In the same year, a hybrid operating room consisting of a mobile O-arm CT scan system (Medtronic Japan Co., Ltd., Tokyo, Japan) was reported by Ohtaka's et al. in Japan [13]. The team managed to conduct localization for small pulmonary nodules in their newly established hybrid suite. Nevertheless, limiting radiation exposure to the patient and its time-consuming characteristic remain to be resolved.

In 2017, Ujiie's group introduced their multiple detector CT (MDCT) (Definition FLASH; Siemens, Washington, DC, USA) system assembled within a hybrid operating room [14]. With the assistance of the novel minimally invasive near-infrared thoracoscopic technique, they successfully localized small lung nodules of the patient. Although the imaging of the target lesion and the surgery were conducted in the same hybrid operating room, the possibility of wire dislocation and complication caused by patient transfer was not decreased.

Chao et al. also in 2017 described an imaging guided thoracoscopic resection of a ground-glass opacity lesion by percutaneous hookwire localization, which is performed in a hybrid operating room equipped with a robotic C-arm CT (Artis zeego,

Artis zeego multi-axis robotic imaging system (Siemens Healthcare AG, Forchheim, Germany) with PURE™ Platform
Free-floating Artis OR table
Large display mounted on rails
syngo X Workplace (Siemens Healthcare AG, Forchheim, Germany)
Steris OR lamps
Dräger anesthetic workplace & Dräger Motiva supply unit
Olympus and Karl-Storz endoscopic systems with near-infrared capabilities
Medtronic SuperDimension™ navigation system (Covidien, Minneapolis, MN, USA)
Emprint™ Microwave Ablation System (Medtronic, USA)
2.5 m × 2.5 m (8.2 ft × 8.2 ft) laminar airflow field

Table 1.
Configurations of the hybrid operation room (OR) (Prince of Wales Hospital, Hong Kong).

Year	Authors	Imaging device
2013	Bueno et al. [11]	CBCT, MRI, PET, near-infrared imaging
2014	Ng et al. [12]	Robotic C-arm CBCT
2014	Ohtaka et al. [13]	O-arm CT
2017	Ujiie et al. [14]	Multiple detector CT (MDCT)
2017	Chao et al. [15]	Robotic C-arm CBCT

Table 2.
Summary of recently reported hybrid OR for image-guided thoracic surgery.

Siemens Healthcare GmbH, Erlangen, Germany) system [15]. The C-arm CT is considered better than MDCT and O-arm CT because of its flexibility and ability to perform circumferential scanning around the surgical table. However, there are still several limits of the single-stage approach, such as the availability of the high-cost hybrid OR, the time-consuming and complicated repositioning of the C-arm instrument, and the risk of air embolism because of needle placement (**Table 2**) [16].

3. Current needs in thoracic surgery

With the popularization of lung screening by chest computed tomography (CT), the detection rate of pulmonary nodules continues to rise [17]. According to a previous study by Gill, for about 8–51% of patients screened on a CT scan, it is unclear that whether their detected pulmonary nodules are benign or malignant [18]. Since early detection and subsequent treatment for lung cancer can reduce mortality [19], the efficient and rapid identification of the nodules' nature has become an increasing challenge for both thoracic clinicians and researchers. Despite the emergence of many innovative techniques which can potentially assist in the diagnosis of pulmonary nodules, the most reliable diagnosing method is surgical excision biopsy with pathological section [20]. Compared with conventional multiport VATS or open biopsy procedure, single-port video-assisted thoracoscopic surgery (VATS) can provide a less invasive way to the resection of pulmonary nodules [3, 6]. However, there are some inherent drawbacks in SPVATS. First, the single-port approach increases the difficulty in localizing the target lesion with limited access for finger palpation

[10] and surgical instrument manipulation within a small incision [21]. Palpating a small lung lesion via minimally invasive access wounds is especially challenging when the lesion is located in a spot far from the pleural surface or it consists of part-solid component with high ground-glass opacity (GGO) [22].

Several techniques have been developed to aid the identification of lung nodules. The conventional two-stage approach for localization of pulmonary nodules includes two steps: image guided preoperative adjunctive localization of the lesion such as hookwire/microcoil implantation or dye marking, and subsequent resection of the nodule in a surgery suite [23]. However, in the procedure of metallic implantation, the metallic bar or hookwire may dislocate during the transfer of the patient to the OR or during the surgical procedure. The lung deflation or the retraction of the wire by the operator can also cause the displacement of the marker [22]. As for dye marking, the diffusion of the dye contrast over time will increase the risk of failure localization. In addition, allergy and embolism are two important side effects of this localizing method which may cause serious consequences [24]. The application of a hybrid operating room can implement the localization and therapeutic procedure within a single room, which can not only save time and cost, but also reduce the rate of pneumothorax, marker dislocation, and dye diffusion [25].

4. Localization via percutaneous approach

As mentioned above, many localization techniques have been developed to help thoracic surgeons with navigation to the pulmonary nodules. By combining the imaging method with adjunctive instruments, such as hookwire or dye marking, the target lesion can be marked in different ways. The family of localization markers can be classified as two types: physical markers, such as hookwire and metallic fiducials, and chemical markers, such as dye marking and radionuclide labeling.

4.1 Hookwire and metallic markers

As the most commonly used localization method for small pulmonary lesions, hookwire has a place in thoracic surgery because of its high success rate [26–28]. Hookwires have long been used in marking breast lesions and relatively solid breast tissues. It was then applied to pulmonary nodules localization by radiologists and thoracic surgeons inspired by its success in treating breast diseases [29]. In a conventional preoperative localization approach, the hookwire is usually inserted into the chest at a radiology suite a few hours before the surgery to facilitate lung nodule localization; however, problems remain such as hookwire migration, pneumothorax, hemothorax, patient discomfort, and potential cost due to the patient transfer between different suites [30]. According to a recent study by Yasufuku et al., around 24% of the patients that underwent hookwire implantation would suffer from pneumothorax. Likewise, the metallic markers are usually implanted before the procedure through percutaneous path and detected by intraoperative fluoroscopy, or occasionally may be palpated [31, 32]. They have the same drawbacks as hookwires (post-procedural pain, pneumothorax, hemothorax, air embolus). When the hookwire or the metallic marker insertion is performed within the hybrid OR setting, their potential complications and risks can be minimized by reducing transfer time which equals "at risk" time for those complications to develop (**Figure 1**). The authors' team has developed a treatment paradigm for small nodules or those with GGO components, known as image guided single-port VATS (iSPVATS) [7]. In their approach, the discussed disadvantages of metallic markers are decreased due to a shortened delay between the localization and the surgery.

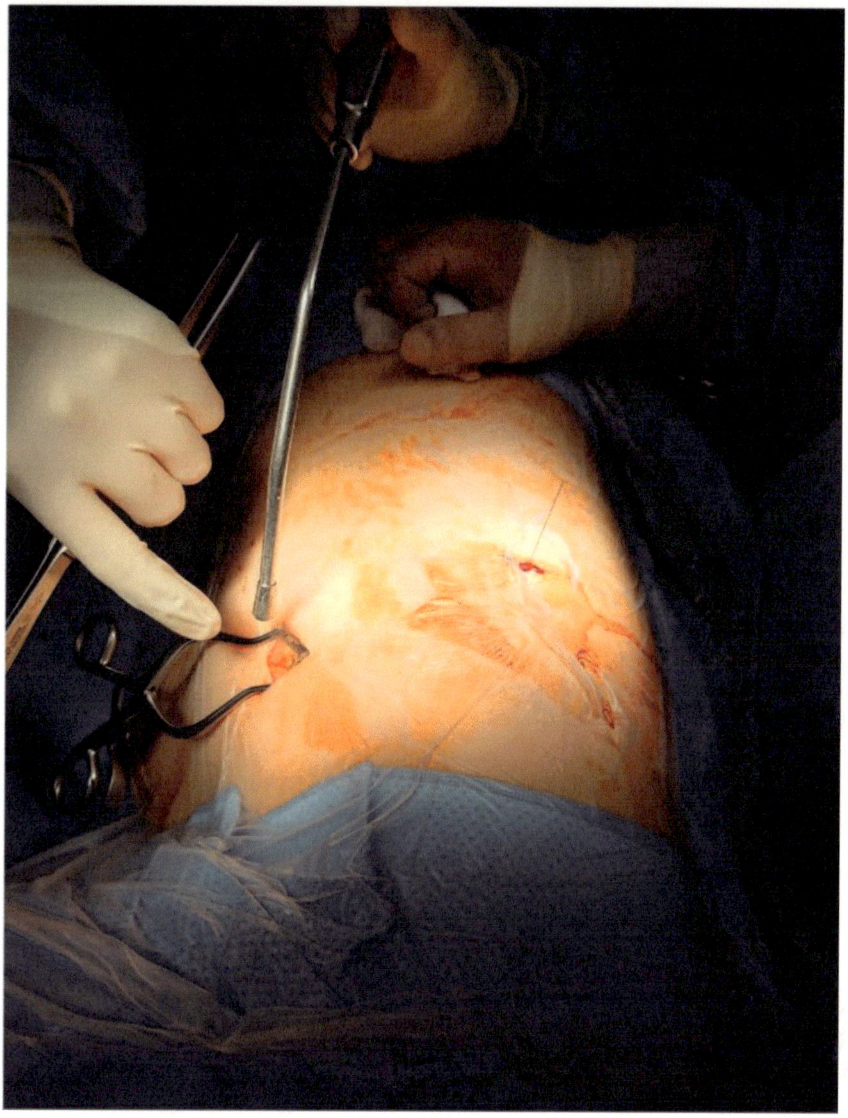

Figure 1.
Patient undergoing uniportal VATS lung resection following posterior hookwire placement in hybrid operating room.

Moreover, if the marker dislodgement happens accidentally, the real-time imaging ability of the hybrid OR allows for a salvage CT scan to be performed to re-localize the target spot.

4.2 Dye marker

Different from hookwire, the dye markers, including methylene blue, barium sulfate, lipiodol and others, are normally injected into the tumor region to help the surgeons localize the lesion usually via either direct vision through a white-light thoracoscopy or fluoroscopy [22]. This marking method also has pleural complications due to the invasive percutaneous approach; besides, it can also be affected by the diffusion of the dye into the parenchyma, and spillage into the pleural cavity leading to difficulty or failure of localization for surgery. More recently, indocyanine green (ICG) has been used as a dye, particularly for deeper lesions as the fluorescence using near infra-red light thoracoscopy could be seen up to 2 cm from pleura. Numerous methods have been described to reduce diffusion of dye into parenchyma over time, include mixing the dye with albumin, biological glue or lipiodol. Other important issues of the percutaneous dye approach are possible allergy and air embolism during the injection of the dye marking which may cause serious and even life-threatening sequelae. An early study on 25 patients undergoing image-guided percutaneous dye localization in the hybrid OR was reported by a group in Taiwan [33]. During the procedure, cone-beam CT was applied for the confirmation of the successful injection. Nevertheless, the drawbacks described before, though rare could still occur; and furthermore, nodules that are located near the apex, diaphragm and mediastinum are often difficult or risky to approach from percutaneous route.

5. Localization via endobronchial approach

5.1 Electromagnetic navigation bronchoscopy (ENB)

Electromagnetic navigation bronchoscopy (ENB) is a superior bronchoscopic technique utilizing electromagnetic sensor technology to facilitate the navigation of the probe to the target region [34]. The typical technological process of an ENB-assisted biopsy or marking includes:

1. Navigational stage implemented by "electromagnetic sensor technology in combination with virtual three-dimensional (3D) bronchial reconstruction of CT images that can be paired with the true bronchoscopic images" [34].

2. The lock of extended working channel (EWC) after successful navigation and withdrawing the sensor tip.

3. The delivery of different tools for biopsy or marking the lesions.

Over the last ten years or so, this approach has been developed into a powerful tool for localization and following diagnosis of the peripheral pulmonary lesions [35]. Success rate of nodule localization can be as high as 93% when combining ENB with endobronchial ultrasound [36]. Nevertheless, identifying a small lesion with a high GGO component can be a challenging task for ENB with adjunctive methods such as endobronchial ultrasound and standard fluoroscopy [5]. To improve the performance of ENB-related techniques, the author's group developed an innovative paradigm which combines the ENB with cone-beam computed tomography (CBCT) [37] (**Figure 2**). The steps of this new approach are as following:

1. Standard ENB-guided localization.

2. Anchoring of EWC.

3. Switch-off of ENB system.

4. Activation of CBCT.

5. A 6-second CBCT scan allows visualization of the target lesion, adjacent structures, and the relative position of the EWC and tools.

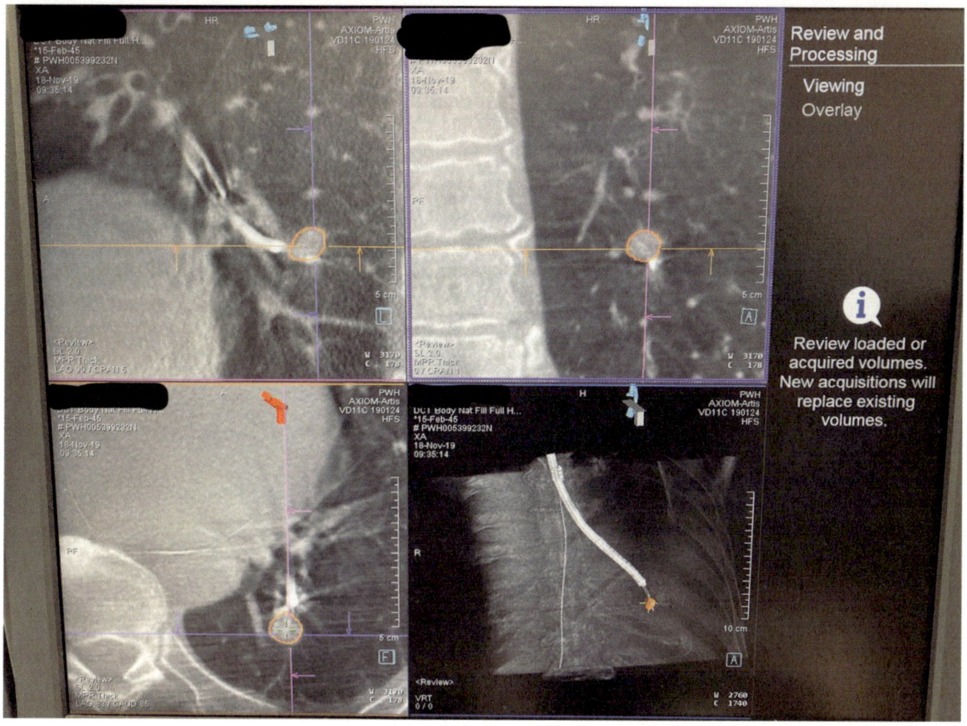

Figure 2.
Cone-beam CT images from hybrid OR showing successful left lower lobe 9 mm nodule electromagnetic navigation bronchoscopy biopsy guided by cone-beam computed tomography scan and assistance from PURE™ platform segmentation software.

Notably, two CBCT scans during the procedure would provide the best outcomes: the first CBCT is the pre-procedure scan that provides the latest information on positional relation of the lesion to allow software (such as i-guide, Siemens, Germany) to mark your lesion, while the second CBCT is for confirming whether the biopsy tool or marker has been deployed in the right position. This technique has been applied on 12 patients with nodules from 8 mm to 39 mm. There is no complication found, and the diagnostic rate was 83.3% [38].

5.2 Metallic marker

The utilization of ENB has been broadened in recent years to encompass enabling adjunctive therapies and direct therapies. Apart from the navigation system for biopsy, it can also be used to assist in the placement of different kinds of markers. Fiducials are dense markers made of gold or platinum, and they are often used for simultaneous tumor tracking due to its imaging characteristics, to aid in specialized targeted radiotherapies and surgery, in particularly for lesion localization. Anantham's group reported ENB-guided insertion of 39 metallic fiducials into 9 patients for robotic stereotactic radiosurgery of lung tumors. Not surprisingly, dislodgement is one of the major problems of this approach [39]. In addition, the small risk of allergic reaction and complications arising from the prolonged duration of implantation of these markers are also issues to be considered when placing these markers.

5.3 Dye marker

Apart from metallic materials, dye markers have also been developed as a combination with ENB for localization of lung nodules. Bolton et al. reported dye

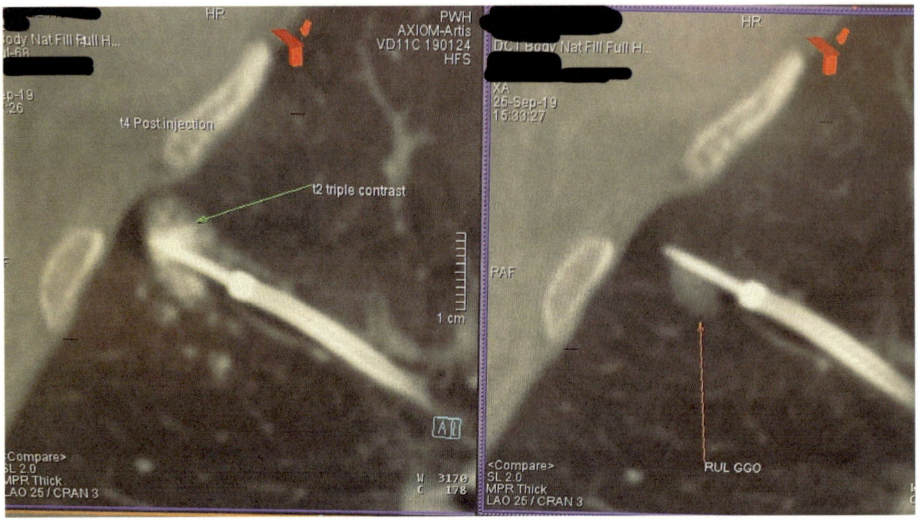

Figure 3.
Cone-beam CT images of dye marking of right upper lobe 7 mm nodule for surgical resection. The right image is the deployed injection needle before injection of dye while the left image is the CT immediately after injection of dye.

marking via ENB under fluoroscopic assistance for 19 subjects. In this case, methylene blue was injected into the target lesion, and the use of intraoperative fluoroscopy is required as confirmation of a successful localization [40]. Dye marker injection by ENB in the hybrid operating room setting can lead to a lower risk of dye diffusion as the time interval between injection and surgery can be reduced.

In 2016, Marino et al. studied ENB-guided trans-bronchial dye injection followed by VATS sublobar resection [41]. Among all the 72 lung nodules ranging from 4 mm to 17 mm, 70 were identified successfully. Notably, an extra shot of methylene blue was injected to the pleura once it is confirmed that the distance between the nodule and the surface of the pleura is over 4 mm. It is believed that the application of hybrid OR technique will improve the success rate of dye placement and enables the precise visualization of the margin of the tumor [41].

In recent years, the fluorescent dye indocyanine green (ICG) has been applied in medical research including optical mapping of cardiac activity, measurements of liver blood flow and ophthalmology [42, 43]. In 2018, Wen's team reported their ICG marking in the hybrid OR for 26 patients with pulmonary nodules [44]. The ICG can remain at the target spot for more than six hours in vivo, and the near-infrared (NIR) light thoracoscopy can detect the dye's wavelength without being affected by the color change of the visceral pleura due to anthracosis (**Figure 3**). Also, it will not influence the result of the pathological examination. Similar to other dye markers, risk of diffusion is one limitation of ICG, as well as specific requirement for NIR device.

6. Bronchoscopic ablation

Lung cancer can be divided into small cell lung cancer (SCLC) and non-small cell lung cancer (NSCLC), among which nearly 80% are NSCLCs [45]. Surgical resection is the gold standard treatment for resectable early stage NSCLCs [46]; however, thermal ablation is considered a safe, cost-effective and ultra-minimally invasive treatment for patients with small tumors who are not suitable for surgery [53]. Thermal or energy-based ablation of tumors means "the local application of extreme temperatures to cause irreversibly pathological cell injury, tumor apoptosis and coagulative necrosis". Catheter-based alternative therapies include radiofrequency ablation (RFA), microwave ablation (MWA), and cryoablation (CRA). Among the thermal therapies, RFA and MWA are most commonly used for lung cancer as alternative approaches.

The most popular approach for ablation has been percutaneous. More recently, bronchoscopic approach to ablation has increasingly been accepted as an alternative to percutaneous approach. Bronchoscopic ablation has advantages over percutaneous of having less complications of pneumothorax and pulmonary-pleural fistula, as well as being scarless. The use of the hybrid OR and CBCT allows the confirmation of appropriate bronchoscopic navigation and positioning of the ablation catheter, calculation of the predicted ablation zone, monitoring of ablation progress, and assessment of the final ablated zone. Thus, for the foreseeable future, CBCT like image quality is critical to enable this form of bronchoscopic catheter therapeutic intervention.

6.1 Radiofrequency ablation (RFA)

In a radiofrequency ablation, one or more radiofrequency electrodes are placed into the tumor under the guidance of computed tomography or ultrasound. A high-frequency alternating current produced by the electrodes can generate 60–100°C temperature by inducing frictional heating in tissues [47]. It is reported that in most recently published RFA cases, conscious sedation or general anesthesia, and no less than 24 h postoperative observation are required. Depending on the size and shape of the tumor, the adjacent normal lung tissue might be burned during the process [48].

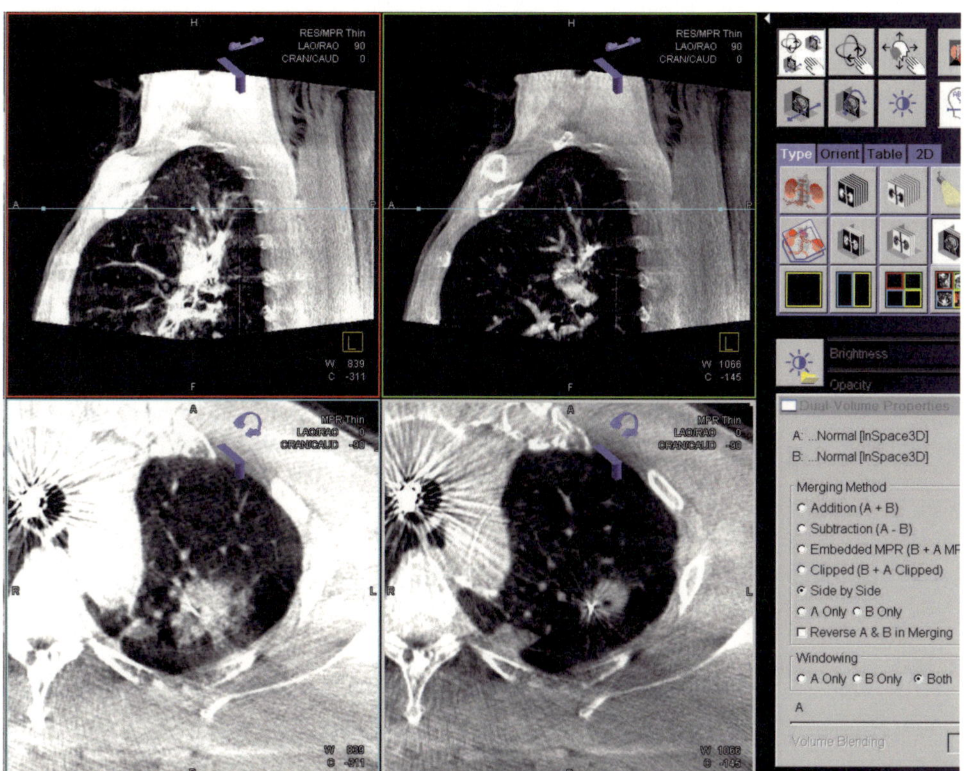

Figure 4.
Cone-beam CT images showing left upper lobe adenocarcinoma bronchoscopically ablated by microwave energy. The right images show the Emprint™ catheter within the tumor before ablation while the left images show CT performed 10 min post ablation.

Because of the mechanism of radiofrequency ablation, the feasibility of this catheter-based approach is determined by the electrical conductance of the target organ. Since the normal lung tissues have a poor electrical conductance and a higher impedance than lung tumors, most current generated by the electrodes will pass through the tumor [49]. Moreover, a phenomenon called "heat sink effect" is another limitation of RFA, which happens when heat absorbed by blood flow or air is carried away from the ablated region, leading to a loss of temperature and decreased RFA efficacy [50, 51].

6.2 Microwave ablation (MWA)

Similar to RFA, MWA utilizes electromagnetic waves to cause localized hyperthermia and induce cell injury and death. During an MWA procedure, heat is generated by the oscillation of electromagnetic field between active dipoles at the tip of MW antennas, causing following realignment and agitation of water molecules and increased kinetic energy. With much higher frequencies compared with RF, electromagnetic radiation is not largely influenced by tissue impedance. As a result, MWA is considered as a more powerful and predictable thermal approach for lung tumors [52]. In a study by Han et al., 28 elderly patients (over 75 years old) with stage I or lymph node-negative stage IIA underwent MWA [53]. As the result shows, the local recurrence rate was 32.1%, and no significant difference was found between the outcome of MWA and RFA. As a limited amount of data available on comparative studies on this topic, further research is needed to evaluate the efficacy of MWA and RFA (**Figure 4**).

7. One-stop-shop: "value" and costs of hybrid OR

As a surgical workspace that integrates imaging devices with a multifunctional surgical table, hybrid OR can provide unparallel imaging support for a variety of surgical scenarios. This one-stop-shop hybrid OR can help with the localization and biopsy of suspected pulmonary nodules in a more efficient and time-saving way. In contrast to conventional approaches, a hybrid OR can provide real-time imaging and increase the success rate for a hookwire insertion or ENB, and also functions as an adjunct in the intraprocedural ultrasonography technique during single-port VATS. In a CT-guided injection of dye makers (barium or lipiodol) within a hybrid OR, the delay between the adjunct placement and the surgery is shorter, minimizing the potential risk of percutaneous complications and diffusion [27]. ENB-guided therapeutic methods such as RFA and MWA provide a safe and effective option for patients with early-stage NSCLCs. Overall, the utilization of hybrid OR on diagnosis, staging, and treating the lung-related diseases has been gaining more and more popularity.

The costs of a hybrid OR depends on the country and institution-specific operational and manual cost. As there is lacking data and knowledge on this issue, future investigations are needed to compare approaches conducted within hybrid OR and those through conventional multi-stop multi-shop means.

8. Future developments of hybrid OR

The hybrid operating room is progressively used in the thoracic surgery to improve the accuracy of the procedures and to provide useful guidance to both endoscopy and surgical procedures. The new era of hybrid thoracic surgery does not depend only on its imaging superiority but also the integration of other technologies, including 3D printing, robotic bronchoscopy and NOTES lung surgery, just to name a few. The application of the precise imaging provided by the real-time cone-beam computed tomography will be greatly improved as a result of the development of adjunct related technologies.

The hybrid operating room with real-time cone-beam computed tomography can be combined with 3D printing to provide precise customization of prostheses. This facility can provide images of post-resection chest wall defects which can be used for 3D image reconstruction and segmentation to generate an accurate stereo vision of the chest wall defect. The immediate transfer of data for 3D printing within the operating room could make the process of surgery more tailored by custom 3D printing prostheses for that specific defect and stature of the patient.

Recently, the number of navigational bronchoscopy or catheter-based platforms is increasing rapidly which will enable more accurate navigation and will improve the safety and efficacy of the operation. The hybrid operating room can provide precise imaging support to the implementation of these technologies which is of vital importance because the positioning of lesions is the foundation for conducting surgery and its accuracy will provide guidance to the specific operational technologies. Furthermore, these platforms will promote the main use of navigational bronchoscopy in the hybrid operating room at the same time which means more precise localization of the lesions. The combination of robotic bronchoscopy with the hybrid operating room may further enhance localization accuracy and allow thoracic surgery with greater precision.

It is said that the natural orifice transluminal endoscopic surgery (NOTES) platforms and single incision robotic platforms will become the next generation of tools for performing uniportal VATS and incisionless "surgery" enabling further reduction in access trauma and more surgical precision. Some of the short comings of current NOTES platforms could be at least in part be addressed by using high precision imaging from hybrid operation room for localization, assisting the surgery and confirming efficacy of the procedure.

In summary, it is anticipated that the hybrid operating room will play a more and more important role in image-guided thoracic surgery as it establishes an efficient and integrated procedural flow for the operation process. It can be combined with many promising technologies to achieve the accurate control of the endoscopic and surgical procedure. More advanced modalities of imaging could be further incorporated in to this set up to provide additional imaging information and precise details which will lead us to a safer and more meticulous surgery of the future.

Acknowledgements

This work is partly supported by the Academic Equipment Grant (AEG) Project codes 3029988; 3029992; 3029993 (2018/19), from the Chinese University of Hong Kong; and Research Grants Council (RGC) Grant 2019/20; Project reference no: 14119019.

Conflict of interest

EQY has no conflicts of interest. CSHN is a consultant for Siemens Healthineers, Medtronic and Johnson and Johnson.

Notes/thanks/other declarations

Nil.

Author details

Evan Qize Yuan and Calvin Sze Hang Ng*
Division of Cardiothoracic Surgery, Department of Surgery, Prince of Wales Hospital, The Chinese University of Hong Kong, Hong Kong SAR

*Address all correspondence to: calvinng@surgery.cuhk.edu.hk

References

[1] Ng CS, Gonzalez-Rivas D, D'Amico TA, Rocco G. Uniportal VATS—A new era in lung cancer surgery. Journal of Thoracic Disease. 2015;**7**(8):1489-1491. DOI: 10.3978/j.issn.2072-1439.2015.08.19

[2] Zhao ZR, Ng CSH. Hookwire localization of pulmonary nodules in uniportal VATS. In: Atlas of Uniportal Video Assisted Thoracic Surgery. Singapore: Springer; 2019. pp. 95-99. DOI: 10.1007/978-981-13-2604-2_14

[3] Ng CS, Lau KK, Gonzalez-Rivas D, Rocco G. Evolution in surgical approach and techniques for lung cancer. Thorax. 2013;**68**:681. DOI: 10.1136/thoraxjnl-2012-203157

[4] Ng CS, Rocco G, Wong RH, Lau RW, Yu SC, Yim AP. Uniportal and single-incision video-assisted thoracic surgery: The state of the art. Interactive Cardiovascular and Thoracic Surgery. 2014;**19**:661-666. DOI: 10.1093/icvts/ivu200

[5] Zhao ZR, Li Z, Situ DR, Ng CS. Recent clinical innovations in thoracic surgery in Hong Kong. Journal of Thoracic Disease. 2016;**8**(Suppl 8): S618-S626. DOI: 10.21037/jtd.2016.03.93

[6] Ng CS. Uniportal VATS in Asia. Journal of Thoracic Disease. 2013;**5**:S221-S225

[7] Ng CS, Man Chu C, Kwok MW, Yim AP, Wong RH. Hybrid DynaCT scan-guided localization single-port lobectomy [corrected]. Chest. 2015;**147**:e76-e78

[8] Zhao ZR, Lau RW, Yu PS, Wong RH, Ng CS. Image-guided localization of small lung nodules in video-assisted thoracic surgery. Journal of Thoracic Disease. 2016;**8**(Suppl 9):S731-S737. DOI: 10.21037/jtd.2016.09.47

[9] Zhao ZR, Lau RW, Yu PS, Ng CS. Devising the guidelines: The techniques of pulmonary nodule localization in uniportal video-assisted thoracic surgery—Hybrid operating room in the future. Journal of Thoracic Disease. 2019. DOI: 10.21037/jtd.2019.01.82

[10] Saleh WK, Abu OAJ, Lumsden A, Ramchandani MK. Simultaneous localization and removal of lung nodules through extended use of the hybrid suite. Methodist DeBakey Cardiovascular Journal. 2015;**11**(4): 245-246. DOI: 10.14797/mdcj-11-4-245

[11] Advanced Multimodality Image Guided Operating (AMIGO). 2016. Available from: http://www.brighamandwomens.org/research/amigo/default.aspx [Accessed: 01 September 2018]

[12] Zhao ZR, Ng CSH. Image-guided uniportal VATS in the hybrid operating room. In: Atlas of Uniportal Video Assisted Thoracic Surgery. Singapore: Springer; 2019. pp. 269-278. DOI: 10.1007/978-981-13-2604-2_39

[13] Ohtaka K, Takahashi Y, Kaga K, et al. Video-assisted thoracoscopic surgery using mobile computed tomography: New method for locating of small lung nodules. Journal of Cardiothoracic Surgery. 2014;**9**:110

[14] Ujiie H, Kato T, Hu HP, et al. A novel minimally invasive near-infrared thoracoscopic localization technique of small pulmonary nodules: A phase I feasibility trial. The Journal of Thoracic and Cardiovascular Surgery. 2017;**154**:702-711

[15] Hsieh CP, Hsieh MJ, Fang HY, Chao YK. Imaging-guided thoracoscopic resection of a ground-glass opacity lesion in a hybrid operating room equipped with a robotic C-arm CT system. Journal of Thoracic Disease.

2017;**9**(5):E416-E419. DOI: 10.21037/jtd.2017.04.48

[16] Freund MC, Petersen J, Goder KC, et al. Systemic air embolism during percutaneous core needle biopsy of the lung: Frequency and risk factors. BMC Pulmonary Medicine. 2012;**12**:2

[17] Team NLSTR, Aberle DR, Adams AM, Berg CD, Black WC, Clapp JD, et al. Reduced lung-cancer mortality with low-dose computed tomographic screening. The New England Journal of Medicine. 2011;**365**:395-409

[18] Gill RR, Jaklitsch MT, Jacobson FL. Controversies in lung cancer screening (internet). Journal of the American College of Radiology. 2013;**10**:931-936

[19] Team NLSTR, Church TR, Black WC, et al. Results of initial low-dose computed tomographic screening for lung cancer. The New England Journal of Medicine. 2013;**368**:1980-1991

[20] Chow SC, Ng CS. Recent developments in video-assisted thoracoscopic surgery for pulmonary nodule management. Journal of Thoracic Disease. 2016;**8**(Suppl 6): S509-S516. DOI: 10.21037/jtd.2016.03.18

[21] Ng CS, Pickens A, Siegel JM, et al. A novel narrow profile articulating powered vascular stapler provides superior access and haemostasis equivalent to conventional devices. European Journal of Cardio-Thoracic Surgery. 2016;**49**(Suppl 1):i73-i78

[22] Zhao ZR, Lau RW, Ng CS. Hybrid theatre and alternative localization techniques in conventional and single-port video-assisted thoracoscopic surgery. Journal of Thoracic Disease. 2016;**8**(Suppl 3):S319-S327. DOI: 10.3978/j.issn.2072-1439.2016.02.27

[23] Chao Y-K, Pan K-T, Wen C-T, Fang H-Y, Hsieh M-J. A comparison of efficacy and safety of preoperative versus intraoperative computed tomography-guided thoracoscopic lung resection. The Journal of Thoracic and Cardiovascular Surgery. 2018;**156**(5):1974-1983. DOI: 10.1016/j.jtcvs.2018.06.088

[24] Watanabe K, Nomori H, Ohtsuka T, et al. Usefulness and complications of computed tomography-guided lipiodol marking for fluoroscopy-assisted thoracoscopic resection of small pulmonary nodules: Experience with 174 nodules. The Journal of Thoracic and Cardiovascular Surgery. 2006;**132**:320-324

[25] Zhao Z-R, Lau RWH, Ng CSH. Hybrid theater and uniportal video-assisted thoracic surgery. Thoracic Surgery Clinics. 2017;**27**(4):347-355. DOI: 10.1016/j.thorsurg.2017.06.003

[26] Chen Y-R, Yeow K-M, Lee J-Y, Su IH, Chu S-Y, Lee C-H, et al. CT-guided hook wire localization of sub- pleural lung lesions for video-assisted thoracoscopic surgery (VATS). Journal of the Formosan Medical Association. 2007;**106**:911-918

[27] Klinkenberg TJ, Dinjens L, Wolf RFE, van der Wekken AJ, van de Wauwer C, de Bock GH, et al. CT-guided percutaneous hookwire localization increases the efficacy and safety of VATS for pulmonary nodules. Journal of Surgical Oncology. 2017;**115**:898-904

[28] Ichinose J, Kohno T, Fujimori S, Harano T, Suzuki S. Efficacy and complications of computed tomography-guided hook wire localization. The Annals of Thoracic Surgery. 2013;**96**:1203-1208

[29] Kothapalli PR, Wyler von Ballmoos MC, Chinnadurai P,

Lumsden AB, Ramchandani MK. Value of the hybrid operating theater for an integrated approach to diagnosis and treatment of pulmonary nodules in 2019. Frontiers in Surgery. 2019;**6**:36. DOI: 10.3389/fsurg.2019.00036

[30] Ciriaco P, Negri G, Puglisi A, Nicoletti R, Del Maschio A, Zannini P. Video-assisted thoracoscopic surgery for pulmonary nodules: Rationale for preoperative computed tomography-guided hookwire localization. European Journal of Cardio-Thoracic Surgery. 2004;**25**:429-433. DOI: 10.1016/j.ejcts.2003.11.036

[31] Miyoshi T, Kondo K, Takizawa H, et al. Fluoroscopy- assisted thoracoscopic resection of pulmonary nodules after computed tomography-guided bronchoscopic metallic coil marking. The Journal of Thoracic and Cardiovascular Surgery. 2006;**131**:704-710

[32] Mayo JR, Clifton JC, Powell TI, et al. Lung nodules: CT-guided placement of microcoils to direct video-assisted thoracoscopic surgical resection. Radiology. 2009;**250**:576-585

[33] Yang SM, Ko WC, Lin MW, et al. Image-guided thoracoscopic surgery with dye localization in a hybrid operating room. Journal of Thoracic Disease. 2016;**8**(Suppl 9):S681-S689

[34] Schwarz Y, Mehta AC, Ernst A, et al. Electromagnetic navigation during flexible bronchoscopy. Respiration. 2003;**70**:516-522

[35] Chee A, Stather DR, Maceachern P, et al. Diagnostic utility of peripheral endobronchial ultrasound with electromagnetic navigation bronchoscopy in peripheral lung nodules. Respirology. 2013;**18**:784-789

[36] Eberhardt R, Anantham D, Herth F, et al. Electromagnetic navigation diagnostic bronchoscopy in peripheral lung lesions. Chest. 2007;**131**:1800-1805

[37] Ng CS, Yu SC, Lau RW, Yim AP. Hybrid DynaCT-guided electromagnetic navigational bronchoscopic biopsy†. European Journal of Cardio-Thoracic Surgery. 2016;**49**:i87-i88

[38] Lau WH, Chow CYS, Ho YKJ, et al. Hybrid operating room DynaCT real-time image guided electromagnetic navigation bronchoscopic biopsy (iENB)—The initial experience. Respirology. 2016;**21**(Suppl 3):74

[39] Anantham D, Feller-Kopman D, Shanmugham LN, et al. Electromagnetic navigation bronchoscopy-guided fiducial placement for robotic stereotactic radiosurgery of lung tumors: A feasibility study. Chest. 2007;**132**:930-935

[40] Bolton WD, Howe H 3rd, Stephenson JE. The utility of electromagnetic navigational bronchoscopy as a localization tool for robotic resection of small pulmonary nodules. The Annals of Thoracic Surgery. 2014;**98**:471-475. discussion 475-6

[41] Rocco R, Rocco G. Future study direction on single port (uniportal) VATS. Journal of Thoracic Disease. 2016;**8**:S328-S332

[42] Yannuzzi LA. Indocyanine green angiography: A perspective on use in the clinical setting. American Journal of Ophthalmology. 2011;**151**:745-51.e1

[43] Zelken JA, Tufaro AP. Current trends and emerging future of Indocyanine green usage in surgery and oncology: An update. Annals of Surgical Oncology. 2015;**22**(Suppl 3):S1271-S1283

[44] Wen CT, Liu YY, Fang HY, et al. Image-guided video-assisted thoracoscopic small lung tumor resection using near-infrared marking. Surgical Endoscopy. 2018;**32**:4673-4680

[45] Non-Small Cell Lung Cancer Treatment (PDQ®)–Patient Version. n.d. Available from: https://www.cancer.gov/types/lung/patient/non-small-cell-lung-treatment-pdq

[46] Ng CS, Zhao ZR, Lau RW. Tailored therapy for stage I non-small-cell lung cancer. Journal of Clinical Oncology. 2017;**35**:268-270

[47] Chu KF, Dupuy DE. Thermal ablation of tumours: Biological mechanisms and advances in therapy. Nature Reviews Cancer. 2014;**14**(3):199-208. DOI: 10.1038/nrc3672

[48] Zhao ZR, Lau RW, Ng CS. Catheter-based alternative treatment for early-stage lung cancer with a high-risk for morbidity. Journal of Thoracic Disease. 2018;**10**(Suppl 16):S1864-S1870. DOI: 10.21037/jtd.2018.03.151

[49] Tafti BA, Genshaft S, Suh R, Abtin F. Lung ablation: Indications and techniques. Seminars in Interventional Radiology. 2019;**36**(03):163-175. DOI: 10.1055/s-0039-1693981

[50] Muralidharan V, Malcontenti-Wilson C, Christophi C. Effect of blood flow occlusion on laser hyperthermia for liver metastases. The Journal of Surgical Research. 2002;**103**:165-174

[51] Whelan WM, Wyman DR, Wilson BC. Investigations of large vessel cooling during interstitial laser heating. Medical Physics. 1995;**22**:105-115

[52] Brace CL. Radiofrequency and microwave ablation of the liver, lung, kidney, and bone: What are the differences? (/products/ejournals/linkout/10.1055/s-0039-1693981/id/JR001155-7). Current Problems in Diagnostic Radiology. 2009;**38**(03):135-143

[53] Gage AA, Baust J. Mechanisms of tissue injury in cryosurgery. Cryobiology. 1998;**37**:171-186